Primary Care Ophthalmology

Editor

JOEL J. HEIDELBAUGH

PRIMARY CARE: CLINICS IN OFFICE PRACTICE

www.primarycare.theclinics.com

Consulting Editor
JOEL J. HEIDELBAUGH

September 2015 • Volume 42 • Number 3

ELSEVIER

1600 John F. Kennedy Boulevard • Suite 1800 • Philadelphia, Pennsylvania, 19103-2899

http://www.theclinics.com

PRIMARY CARE: CLINICS IN OFFICE PRACTICE Volume 42, Number 3
September 2015 ISSN 0095-4543, ISBN-13: 978-0-323-39579-3

Editor: Jessica McCool
Developmental Editor: Colleen Viola

Primary Care: Clinics in Office Practice (ISSN: 0095–4543) is published quarterly by Elsevier Inc., 360 Park Avenue South, New York, NY 10010-1710. Months of issue are March, June, September, and December. Periodicals postage paid at New York, NY and additional mailing offices. Subscription prices are $225.00 per year (US individuals), $392.00 (US institutions), $115.00 (US students), $275.00 (Canadian individuals), $444.00 (Canadian institutions), $175.00 (Canadian students), $345.00 (international individuals), $444.00 (international institutions), and $175.00 (international students). Foreign air speed delivery is included in all *Clinics* subscription prices. All prices are subject to change without notice. POSTMASTER: Send address changes to *Primary Care: Clinics in Office Practice*, Elsevier Periodicals Customer Service, 11830 Westline Industrial Drive, St. Louis, MO 63146. Customer Service Health Sciences Division, Subscription Customer Service, 3251 Riverport Lane, Maryland Heights, MO 63043. **Customer Service: 1-800-654-2452 (U.S. and Canada); 314-447-8871 (outside U.S. and Canada). Fax: 314-447-8029. E-mail: journalscustomerservice-usa@elsevier.com (for print support); journalsonlinesupport-usa@elsevier.com (for online support).**

Reprints. For copies of 100 or more, of articles in this publication, please contact the Commercial Reprints Department, Elsevier Inc., 360 Park Avenue South, New York, NY 10010-1710. Tel. 212-633-3874; Fax: 212-633-3820; E-mail: reprints@elsevier.com.

Primary Care: Clinics in Office Practice is covered in *MEDLINE/PubMed (Index Medicus)* and *EMBASE/ Excerpta Medica, Current Contents/Clinical Medicine, and ISI/BIOMED.*

Contributors

CONSULTING EDITOR

JOEL J. HEIDELBAUGH, MD, FAAFP, FACG
Clinical Professor, Departments of Family Medicine and Urology; Clerkship Director, Department of Family Medicine, University of Michigan Medical School, Ann Arbor, Michigan; Ypsilanti Health Center, Ypsilanti, Michigan

AUTHORS

FAHEEM AHMED, MD
Resident Physician, Wills Eye Hospital, Philadelphia, Pennsylvania

XIAOQIN ALEXA LU, MD
Department of Ophthamology, Emory Eye Clinic, Emory University School of Medicine, Atlanta, Georgia

SUSANA A. ALFONSO, MD, MHCM, FAAFP
Director of Academic and Clinical Integration, Assistant Professor, Department of Family and Preventive Medicine, Interim Medical Director, Emory Family Medicine at Dunwoody, Emory University School of Medicine, Dunwoody, Georgia

RIANOT AMZAT, MD, MPH
Chief Resident, Department of Family and Preventive Medicine, Emory University School of Medicine, Atlanta, Georgia

NIKA BAGHERI, MD
Department of Ophthalmology, Wills Eye Hospital, Thomas Jefferson University, Philadelphia, Pennsylvania

CAROLINE DEBENEDICTIS, MD
Department of Pediatric Ophthalmology, Wills Eye Hospital, Philadelphia, Pennsylvania

ANNE L. DUNLOP, MD, MPH
Department of Family and Preventive Medicine, Emory University School of Medicine, Emory University Nell Hodgson Woodruff School of Nursing, Atlanta, Georgia

JAMES P. DUNN, MD
Director, Uveitis Unit, Retina Division, Wills Eye Hospital, Professor of Ophthalmology, Sidney Kimmel Medical College, Thomas Jefferson University, Philadelphia, Pennsylvania

JONIE D. FAWLEY, PA-C, MPAS
Physician Assistant, Department of Family and Preventive Medicine, Emory Family Medicine at Dunwoody, Emory University School of Medicine, Dunwoody, Georgia

BRAD HAL FELDMAN, MD
Attending Physician, Cornea Service, Wills Eye Hospital, Philadelphia, Pennsylvania

MARIA V. GIBSON, MD, PhD
Department of Family Medicine, Emory University, Emory Family Medicine Center, Dunwoody, Georgia

KAMMI B. GUNTON, MD
Department of Pediatric Ophthalmology, Wills Eye Hospital, Philadelphia, Pennsylvania

ANDREW M. HENDRICK, MD
Department of Ophthalmology, Emory University, Emory Eye Center, Atlanta, Georgia

ROBERT JAMES HOUSE, BA
San Juan Bautista School of Medicine, San Juan, Puerto Rico

JULIE L. JOHNSON, MD, FAAFP
Assistant Professor, Department of Family and Preventive Medicine, Emory University School of Medicine, Atlanta, Georgia

AMBAR KULSHRESHTHA, MD, PhD, MPH
Department of Family Medicine, Emory University, Emory Family Medicine Center, Dunwoody, Georgia

NAHEED LAKHANI, MD
Family Medicine Resident, Emory Family Medicine Residency Program, Atlanta, Georgia

ANAND V. MANTRAVADI, MD
Assistant Professor, Glaucoma Service, Wills Eye Hospital, Jefferson Medical College, Philadelphia, Pennsylvania

NICOLLE MARTIN, MD, MPH
Diplomate, American Board of Preventive Medicine; Department of Family and Preventive Medicine, Emory University School of Medicine, Atlanta, Georgia

SONIA MEHTA, MD
Assistant Professor, Vitreoretinal Diseases and Surgery Service, Department of Ophthalmology, Wills Eye Hospital, Thomas Jefferson University Hospital, Philadelphia, Pennsylvania

PRIYA SHARMA, MD
General Ophthalmology Service, Wills Eye Hospital, Philadelphia, Pennsylvania

JAYANTH SRIDHAR, MD
Mid Atlantic Retina, Retina Service, Wills Eye Hospital, Philadelphia, Pennsylvania

JAY THOMPSON, MD
Lowcountry Eye Specialists, Ladson, South Carolina

NEIL VADHAR, MD
Jefferson Medical College of Thomas Jefferson University, Philadelphia, Pennsylvania

BARRY N. WASSERMAN, MD
Department of Pediatric Ophthalmology, Wills Eye Hospital, Philadelphia, Pennsylvania

JILL RAZOR WELLS, MD
Department of Ophthalmology, Emory University School of Medicine, Atlanta, Georgia

Contents

they can present in either acute or chronic forms; the age of the patient, time of year and physical examination findings are paramount to distinguish the different types of conjunctivitis. Distinguishing between acute viral and bacterial conjunctivitis remains difficult. Patients with prolonged symptoms, poor response to initial management, or evidence of severe disease should be referred to ophthalmology for consultation.

Acute vision loss can be transient (lasting <24 hours) or persistent (lasting >24 hours). When patients present with acute vision loss, it is important to ascertain the duration of vision loss and whether it is a unilateral process affecting one eye or a bilateral process affecting both eyes. This article focuses on causes of acute vision loss in the nontraumatic setting and provides management pearls to help health care providers better triage these patients.

Corneal abrasions and corneal foreign bodies are frequently encountered ophthalmological injuries that are commonly diagnosed and managed by primary care physicians. The clinical course of a corneal epithelial defect can range from a relatively benign self-healing abrasion to a potentially sight-threatening complication such as a corneal ulcer, recurrent erosion, or traumatic iritis. A detailed clinical history regarding risk factors and exposure, along with a thorough slit lamp examination with fluorescein dye are essential for proper diagnosis and treatment, as well as to rule out penetrating globe injuries. Referral to an ophthalmologist is recommended in difficult cases or if other injuries are suspected.

Age-related macular degeneration (AMD) is the leading cause of vision loss in the elderly. AMD is diagnosed based on characteristic retinal findings in individuals older than 50. Early detection and treatment are critical in increasing the likelihood of retaining good and functional vision.

Defining the type of strabismus creates a framework for work-up and management. Comitant esotropia is most commonly a childhood condition treated with glasses and surgery. Comitant exotropia is often a childhood condition that may require surgical correction. Microvascular disease is the most common cause of ocular cranial nerve palsies in adult patients.

Cataract surgery with an intraocular lens implant is one of the most common and thought to be the most effective surgical procedure in any field of medicine. Although aging is the most common cause, other factors are also known to be associated with cataract formation. Although cataracts are the domain of ophthalmology, primary care physicians are frequently the ones to whom patients present with vision complaints. Knowledge of cataract symptoms, how to evaluate them, and a basic understanding of the surgery to correct cataracts make primary care physicians an integral part of treating this leading cause of preventable blindness.

Flashes and floaters are common ocular complaints. Flashes refer to aberrations of light that are seen in a patient's field of gaze. The flashes can be of varying sizes, colors, frequency, and durations, depending on the cause. Floaters are another common visual phenomenon caused by particles or debris in the vitreous gel of the eye that cause shadows and thus visual changes, especially against bright backgrounds and in brightly lit environments. Flashes and floaters can occur individually or together. This article discusses common causes of flashes and floaters to help with the triaging and management of these patients.

Glaucoma is a multifactorial degenerative optic neuropathy that can progress at variable rates and afflict all age groups. It is the second leading cause of blindness worldwide. The disease is commonly divided into 2 major subtypes, open angle and angle closure. Diagnosis of glaucoma is made by a combination of identifying characteristic changes of the optic nerve, functional testing such as visual fields, and structural imaging of the optic nerve. Management is aimed at reducing intraocular pressure (IOP). Patients with known risk factors should be referred to an ophthalmologist for complete evaluation.

The prevalence of diabetes is on the rise globally as are the consequences, such as diabetic retinopathy. Diabetic retinopathy is a leading cause of vision loss in working-age adults in developed countries. Visual impairment as a result of diabetic retinopathy has a significant negative impact on the patient's quality of life and their ability to successfully manage their disease. Glycemic control, blood pressure normalization, and lipid management form the basis for long-term diabetes management and protection from worsening eye disease.

PRIMARY CARE:
CLINICS IN OFFICE PRACTICE

RELATED INTEREST

Neuroimaging Clinics, August 2015 (Vol. 25, Issue 3)
Orbit and Neuro-ophthalmic Imaging
Juan E. Gutierrez, *Editor*
Available at: http://www.neuroimaging.theclinics.com/

THE CLINICS ARE AVAILABLE ONLINE!
Access your subscription at:
www.theclinics.com

Foreword

The Complexity of Eye Diseases

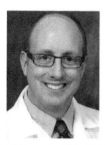

Joel J. Heidelbaugh, MD, FAAFP, FACG
Consulting Editor

Complaints of the eye often scare primary care clinicians. The eyes are vital organs subjected to the perils of chronic diseases and are at a great risk of acute infection and injury that can quickly and permanently compromise their function. Primary care clinicians are generally poorly trained in even basic ophthalmology, so they often feel limited in the approach and diagnosis to many presenting complaints of the eye. Depending on the location of primary care practices, the luxury of an ophthalmologist to evaluate the patient with an ocular complaint in a timely fashion may not always be available.

This issue of *Primary Care: Clinics in Office Practice* explores the wide spectrum of eye diseases encompassing both acute and chronic diseases. The first article provides a detailed introduction to the approach to the patient with a red eye, which is often a common yet concerning presenting complaint in ambulatory care practices. Subsequent articles explore acute conditions, including herpes zoster ophthalmicus, uveitis, conjunctivitis, acute vision loss, and corneal abrasions. Chronic ocular conditions, including macular degeneration, strabismus, cataracts, flashes and floaters, glaucoma, and diabetic retinopathy, are also explored in detail. The importance of augmenting knowledge in these topics cannot be understated, as primary care clinicians can often manage many of these acute conditions, and plays an integral role in the prevention and screening of these chronic conditions.

It was a pleasure to serve as the guest editor for this issue of *Primary Care: Clinics in Office Practice* dedicated to the topic of ophthalmology. I am grateful for the dedicated authors who lent their time, expertise, and wisdom to create informative articles for this compendium of commonly encountered conditions in ambulatory care ophthalmology. Admittedly, I learned more about office-based ophthalmology in reviewing these articles than I did in both medical school and family medicine residency combined! This issue should serve as an invaluable reference for learners of ambulatory care medicine at all levels, but certainly can act as a foundation of "the basics and essentials" of ophthalmology, allowing primary care clinicians to appropriately diagnose and manage

Prim Care Clin Office Pract 42 (2015) ix–x
http://dx.doi.org/10.1016/j.pop.2015.07.001
0095-4543/15/$ – see front matter © 2015 Published by Elsevier Inc.

primarycare.theclinics.com

the spectrum of complexity of common conditions of the eye as well as to refer to an ophthalmologist when an urgency arises.

Joel J. Heidelbaugh, MD, FAAFP, FACG
Departments of Family Medicine and Urology
University of Michigan Medical School
Ann Arbor, MI 48109, USA

Ypsilanti Health Center
200 Arnet Suite 200
Ypsilanti, MI 48198, USA

E-mail address:
jheidel@umich.edu

Approach to Red Eye for Primary Care Practitioners

Anne L. Dunlop, MD, MPH[a],*, Jill Razor Wells, MD[b]

KEYWORDS

- Red eye • Primary care evaluation • Ocular inflammation • Vision

KEY POINTS

- Redness of the eye signifies ocular inflammation and is most commonly attributable to benign conditions readily managed by the primary care provider.
- A careful history and physical examination eliciting key signs and symptoms can readily reveal red flags that indicate the need for higher-level ophthalmologic care.
- Red flags warranting prompt ophthalmologic referral include a red eye with severe pain, visual deficits or loss of acuity, discomfort and nausea, corneal ulceration, and hypopyon or hyphema.

BACKGROUND AND PATHOPHYSIOLOGY

Redness of the eye is a sign of ocular inflammation, resulting from dilatation and/or rupture of blood vessels in the eye. Numerous conditions may result in redness of the eye, including conjunctivitis, blepharitis, canaliculitis, dacryocystitis, episcleritis, scleritis, uveitis, iritis, keratitis, orbital cellulitis, corneal injury, foreign body, chemical burn, subconjunctival hemorrhage, dry eye syndrome, and acute angle-closure glaucoma.[1,2]

The primary care provider is often the first clinician to encounter patients with eye complaints; it is reported that, among eye complaints prompting patients to present for medical care, the red eye is one of the most common.[3,4] Although there are few epidemiologic data to quantify the prevalence of the red eye in primary care, conjunctivitis is the most common cause and is one of the leading indications for antibiotic prescription in primary care.[3,4] Although the costs of conditions that present with red eye to primary care have not been estimated, they are likely substantial because of their common occurrence, the need for diagnostic evaluation and treatment, the cost of pharmaceutical therapies, and loss of time from education and work for children and families.

---

[a] Department of Family & Preventive Medicine, Emory University Schools of Medicine, Emory University Nell Hodgson Woodruff School of Nursing, 1520 Clifton Road, Room 240, Atlanta, GA 30322, USA; [b] Department of Ophthalmology, Emory University School of Medicine, 1365B Clifton Road, NE, Atlanta, GA 30322, USA
* Corresponding author.
E-mail address: amlang@emory.edu

Prim Care Clin Office Pract 42 (2015) 267–284
http://dx.doi.org/10.1016/j.pop.2015.05.002
0095-4543/15/$ – see front matter © 2015 Elsevier Inc. All rights reserved.

In most cases, redness of the eye is caused by benign conditions, such as conjunctivitis, that can be readily managed in the primary care setting. However, there are emergent conditions that present with a red eye. The key to successful management of the red eye in the primary care setting lies in recognizing cases with underlying pathophysiology that require immediate referral to an ophthalmologist for emergent management as well as those cases that are self-limited or readily managed in primary care.[1,2] This article provides an overview of the systematic assessment of patients presenting with a red eye in order to provide guidance for distinguishing those who must be referred immediately to an ophthalmologist versus those whose conditions can be managed in the primary care setting.

ASSESSMENT

The assessment of patients presenting to the primary care setting with a red eye should begin with a thorough history.[1–3,5] As for any presenting complaint, the cardinal questions should be queried in terms of the timing of onset, progression over time, duration of symptoms, periodicity or chronicity, unilateral or bilateral nature, and any associated symptoms. However, given the urgency of identifying chemical and other injuries to the eye, as well as other serious conditions, it is suggested that the following questions be asked in the order as presented later. These questions could also be used to triage and advise patients who call the primary care center with a question about a red eye.

- Was there a chemical exposure, injury, or trauma to the eye? If so, what was the nature of the trauma (with a sharp or blunt object, with small particles, metal on metal?)
  - Any chemical injury to the eye or the structures around the eye (whether caused by an acidic or alkaline agent) should be immediately irrigated with sterile saline or water, then immediately referred for emergent evaluation and management. In the case of a patient calling by phone, the patient should be advised to immediately irrigate the affected eye with water at home and emergently seek ophthalmologic care.
  - Any penetrating injury to the eye or the structures around the eye should be immediately referred for emergent evaluation and management.
- Is pain a prominent symptom? Several conditions of the eye can be associated with varying degrees of pain. Pain or tenderness localized to an area of the lid with associated swelling is characteristic of a stye (hordeolum). Mild pain, often described as scratchiness, is associated with conjunctivitis, blepharitis, and episcleritis. Pain of a more moderate nature is associated with keratitis, uveitis, and scleritis. Severe pain in the eye unilaterally, particularly if associated with tearing of the eye, is typical of a corneal abrasion. Severe pain in the eye unilaterally with associated nausea, vomiting, headache, and decreased vision is a hallmark of acute angle-closure glaucoma and warrants immediate referral to an ophthalmologist.
  - If severe pain or eye pain associated with nausea, vomiting, headache, and decreased vision is present the patient should be immediately referred for emergent evaluation and management.
- Is there a foreign body sensation? A foreign body sensation indicates a process that is affecting the cornea.
- Is there associated photophobia (light sensitivity)? The presence of photophobia in conjunction with a red eye, particularly in the presence of a foreign body

sensation, strongly indicates a corneal process. The presence of photophobia without a foreign body sensation suggests uveitis.

○ If uveitis is suspected, the patient should be immediately referred for emergent evaluation and management.

- Has there been contact lens use? If so, does the patient sleep in contact lenses or use tap water to store the lenses? If the patient does use contact lenses and has red eye accompanied by purulent discharge, be concerned for keratitis and a corneal ulcer.

  ○ If keratitis or corneal ulcer is suspected, the patient should be immediately referred for emergent evaluation and management.

- Is the vision affected? The patient should be asked about perceived visual changes in each eye. In addition, the examiner should perform a visual acuity test (as explained later).

  ○ Be concerned for more serious causes of red eye if the patient reports decreased vision in conjunction with a red eye. However, some serious causes of red eye, such as bacterial keratitis, may not affect the vision.

- Is there discharge from the affected eye? Purulent drainage from the eye that persists throughout the day, in the absence of other signs of keratitis and/or corneal ulcer such as foreign body sensation and photophobia, suggests a bacterial conjunctivitis. In particular, bacterial conjunctivitis should be considered if the discharge is purulent, copious, and forms quickly after wiping it away. Morning crusting of the eye without on-going discharge throughout the day can accompany several less serious conditions, including allergic conjunctivitis, viral conjunctivitis, blepharitis, and dry eye. Chlamydial conjunctivitis should be considered in chronic cases of conjunctivitis lasting greater than 3 months with the presence of conjunctival follicles. There is no need for primary care providers to culture the conjunctival discharge.

  ○ If keratitis or corneal ulcer is suspected because of unilateral redness and purulent discharge in the setting of foreign body sensation with photophobia the patient should be immediately referred for emergent evaluation and management.

- Does the patient have medical comorbidities? A variety of autoimmune disorders have associated eye findings that include redness of the eye. In some cases, autoimmune disorders can be associated with scleritis and/or peripheral ulcerative keratitis causing severe redness and pain. However, autoimmune disorders such as Graves disease, Sjögren syndrome, rheumatoid arthritis, Reiter syndrome, systemic lupus erythematosus, Wegener granulomatosis, relapsing polychondritis, polyarteritis nodosa, and human immunodeficiency virus (HIV) are more often associated with a mild, immunogenic conjunctivitis associated with a chronic, mildly red eye with other ocular symptoms being minimal.[1,3,5] In many cases of autoimmune disorders with ocular findings the diagnosis is already known, but sometimes the red eye is the first or most obvious sign.[5] A full description of these disorders of the immune system that can present with redness of the eye are beyond the scope of this article, but brief descriptions of the ocular features that provide clues to these chronic conditions are given here:

  ○ Graves disease: the characteristic signs of Graves ophthalmopathy are proptosis and periorbital edema. There may or may not be ocular symptoms, which may include mild irritation or retro-orbital discomfort; excessive tearing that is often made worse by exposure to cold air, wind, or bright lights; blurring of vision; or diplopia.[6]

o Sjögren syndrome: this autoimmune disorder is characterized by reduced lacrimal and salivary gland function and leads to the sicca complex (dry eyes and dry mouth) with typical ocular symptoms of dryness, burning, and a scratchy sensation that may worsen as the day goes on; other symptoms are mild pain and redness that is typically bilateral. Dryness of the eye can lead to damage to the conjunctiva and corneal epithelium and can predispose to infection.[7]

o Rheumatoid arthritis: this autoimmune disorder primarily involves the joints, but a range of extra-articular manifestations also occur, including ocular manifestations. The sicca complex is a common component of rheumatoid arthritis. In addition, corneal involvement may involve scleritis and keratitis.[8]

o Reiter syndrome: this reactive autoimmune-mediated monoarticular or oligoarticular arthritis typically follows an infection by several days to weeks. Ocular manifestations can occur, but may not. Most commonly, the associated eye conditions include conjunctivitis and anterior uveitis; less common are episcleritis and scleritis.[9]

o Systemic lupus erythematosus: this autoimmune condition affects the skin, joints, kidneys, lungs, nervous system, serous membranes, and other organs. The eye is frequently involved, with the most common manifestation being those of the dry eye component of the sicca complex. Uncommon or rare ophthalmologic manifestations include episcleritis, scleritis, anterior uveitis, and cotton wool exudates from retinal vasculitis.[10]

o Wegener granulomatosis: this small vessel granulomatous autoimmune vasculitis primarily affects the ears, nose, and throat, as well as the lungs and kidneys. However, there is commonly also eye involvement that ranges from conjunctivitis to corneal ulceration, episcleritis, scleritis, optic neuropathy, nasolacrimal duct obstruction, proptosis, diplopia, retinal vasculitis, and uveitis.[11]

o Relapsing polychondritis: this autoimmune condition primarily affects cartilaginous structures and other structures of the body; primarily the ears, nose, eyes, joints, and respiratory tract. Eye involvement is common and takes several forms. Most characteristic is a localized salmon-pink, fleshy patch of the conjunctiva. Also possible are episcleritis, scleritis, ulcerative keratitis, uveitis, and proptosis.[12]

o Polyarteritis nodosa: this autoimmune necrotizing vasculitis that affects medium and small arteries can have a spectrum of ocular findings ranging from a mild immunogenic conjunctivitis, which is most common, to more severe manifestations that include scleritis, ulcerative keratitis, uveitis, retinal vasculitis, pseudotumor of the orbit, and central retinal artery occlusion associated with temporal arteritis.[13]

o HIV: among patients with a CD4+ T-cell count less than 100/mL, there is a substantial increased risk of retinal microvasculopathy and conjunctival microvasculopathy, as well as cytomegalovirus and varicella-zoster virus infection of the eye, which may present as a red eye.[14]

Subconjunctival hemorrhage can occur in the absence of chronic health conditions and is most commonly caused by straining with coughing, sneezing, constipation, and vomiting as well as mild trauma. However, the presence of chronic health conditions such as diabetes mellitus, hypertension, blood clotting disorders, and the use of anticoagulant and antiplatelet medications increases the risk of development of subconjunctival hemorrhage.[2,3] Subconjunctival hemorrhage is almost always self-limited, unless it is associated with a retrobulbar hemorrhage (an ocular emergency resulting from arterial bleeding in the orbital cavity behind the eye), in which case there is associated severe eye pain and decreased vision unilaterally. Also, diabetes mellitus and hypertension, particularly if they are poorly controlled, are strong risk factors for glaucoma and retinal vascular disease. Recent research supports that patients with diabetes or hypertension have a 48% increased risk of developing open-angle glaucoma compared with adults without those chronic conditions.[15]

- Has the patient had past eye surgeries; this may indicate a postsurgical bleeding or infection that warrants immediate ophthalmologic referral.

After a thorough history is obtained, a careful physical examination should be conducted. In cases in which a chemical injury to the eye is reported, immediate irrigation is performed before examination. The physical examination should include each of the following elements:

- General observation of the patient on entering the room provides clues about the cause of the red eye. Lid and conjunctival processes do not cause photophobia or significant pain, thus the patient unaffected by the ambient light. Patients with viral or allergic conjunctivitis typically have accompanying signs such as rhinorrhea and upper respiratory tract symptoms. In contrast, patients with keratitis, anterior uveitis, scleritis, or angle-closure glaucoma are noticeably uncomfortable or in pain.
- Inspection with pen light or ophthalmoscope should proceed systematically, carefully examining the pupil and anterior chamber of the eye and noting the following:
  - Size, shape, and reactivity of the pupil: in cases of angle-closure glaucoma, the pupil is typically fixed in mid-dilation (approximately 4–5 mm in diameter), but occasionally the pupil is miotic. In cases of corneal abrasion, infectious keratitis, or anterior uveitis the pupil is typically pinpoint in size. In the case of anterior uveitis, a misshapen pupil also may be apparent.
    - In cases of angle-closure glaucoma, the pupil typically is poorly reactive to light. Direct photophobia (when the light is directed into the affected eye) as well as consensual photophobia (when the light is directed into the uninvolved eye) is typical of anterior uveitis.
  - Presence of discharge: purulent discharge is characteristic of bacterial conjunctivitis or bacterial keratitis.
  - Pattern of redness: conjunctivitis (whether bacterial, viral, allergic, or toxic) typically involves diffuse injection of the conjunctival vessels involving both the palpebral and the bulbar conjunctiva. In contrast, ciliary flush, a pattern of redness involving injection of the vessels of the limbus (where the cornea transitions to the sclera) with diminished redness toward the equator of the eye, is an indicator of more serious conditions, including infectious keratitis, anterior uveitis, or angle-closure glaucoma, all of which require immediate referral to ophthalmology. Episcleritis and scleritis are typically localized to 1 quadrant of the globe but may be diffuse.
    - If the redness appears hemorrhagic, rather than a pattern of dilated blood vessels, subconjunctival hemorrhage is likely, which is a self-limited condition but may prompt evaluation for presence and control of diabetes, hypertension, and/or blood clotting disorders or the use of anticoagulant or antiplatelet medications.
  - Presence of corneal lesions: in cases of infectious keratitis, it is common to observe the presence of opacifications (white lesions) of the cornea, which

may be seen without fluorescein. In contrast, corneal abrasions are not characterized by the presence of a corneal opacity; however, under the Wood lamp or cobalt blue lamp, any corneal abrasion or foreign body takes up the dye and appear bright. A branching or dendritic opacity that is enhanced by the addition of fluorescein is characteristic of herpes simplex keratitis. Note that the fluorescein examination is performed by applying 1 to 2 drops of topical ophthalmologic anesthetic to the affected eye, wetting the fluorescein paper with a drop of sterile saline, touching the fluorescein strip to the inferior cul-de-sac of the eye, having the patient blink to evenly disburse the dye, and then observing the eye under a Wood lamp or cobalt blue lamp.

○ Presence of hypopyon or hyphema: the presence of a layer of white blood cells in the anterior chamber, a hypopyon, is associated with sight-threatening infectious keratitis or endophthalmitis; patients with this sign must be seen by an ophthalmologist within hours. Hyphema, a layer of red blood cells in the anterior chamber, could indicate that significant trauma has occurred to the globe and also must be seen within hours by an ophthalmologist.

○ Fluorescein examination: corneal defects, whether from abrasion or ulceration or keratitis, are revealed by staining of the area of corneal defect via uptake of fluorescein dye and examination under a Wood or cobalt blue lamp.

- Measurement of visual acuity of each eye should be performed in any patient with an eye complaint. In the assessment of the red eye, it is not important to document the precise visual acuity but rather to determine whether there has been a change in visual acuity from baseline and/or variability in visual acuity between the affected and nonaffected eyes. Thus, an assessment of near vision in the examination room using a near card is acceptable. This assessment should be done by having the patient hold a specifically designed card at a comfortable distance of approximately 36 cm (14 inches), and having the patient cover 1 eye at a time while testing the other; if the patient normally wears glasses, the vision test should be performed while wearing glasses.

○ A reduction of visual acuity, as determined by near card testing that reveals a reduction in the red eye compared with the unaffected eye, suggests a more serious diagnosis that warrants ophthalmologic evaluation, such as infectious keratitis, anterior uveitis, or angle-closure glaucoma.

- Assessment of extraocular movements should also be performed. Limitation of movement in any of the directions in the setting of a red eye may indicate traumatic orbital injury causing muscular entrapment caused by bony or soft tissue injury and swelling.

DIFFERENTIAL DIAGNOSIS

Common causes of red eye are shown in **Table 1**, along with key symptoms on presentation, distinguishing signs, and key management principles.[1–5,16] **Figs. 1–21** show the appearance of each of these conditions. Many of these conditions are reviewed in more depth in this issue. Grouped together are conditions that are self-limited or typically managed in the primary care setting, followed by those that should be promptly referred to ophthalmology, and those that should be immediately referred to ophthalmology for evaluation and management.

RED FLAGS FOR REFERRAL

The key to the appropriate management of patients presenting with a red eye is recognizing conditions that require further evaluation by an ophthalmologist or emergency

Table 1
Conditions presenting with red eye to the primary care setting

Condition	Appearance	Key Symptoms	Distinguishing Signs	Management
Management in Primary Care				
Allergic conjunctivitis	Fig. 1	Pruritus of eyes bilaterally with redness and watery discharge; typically seasonal with accompanying upper respiratory tract symptoms	Diffusely hyperemic conjunctiva with boggy eyelids and conjunctiva, watery (or sometimes mucoid) discharge bilaterally	Systemic antihistamines or topical ophthalmologic agents such as vasoconstrictors, H-1 receptor blockers, NSAIDs, mast cell stabilizers
Bacterial conjunctivitis	Fig. 2	Soreness of the eye and redness that is typically unilateral, with purulent discharge	Diffusely hyperemic conjunctiva with boggy eyelids and conjunctiva, with purulent discharge	Initiate ophthalmic antibiotics; consult an ophthalmologist for abnormal hosts including neonates, immunocompromised, status post ocular surgery, contact lens users
Viral conjunctivitis	Fig. 3	Mild discomfort typically bilaterally with watery, mucoid discharge	Diffusely hyperemic conjunctiva with slightly swollen lids; watery, mucoid (nonpurulent) discharge, swollen preauricular or submandibular lymph nodes	No treatment required because this is a self-limited condition that resolves within 14 d. Refer only if diagnosis is in question or keratitis is suspected
Blepharitis	Fig. 4	Gritty, burning sensation and matting of eyelashes and lids, especially on awakening	Red, thickened eyelid margins. Mildly red, flaky eyelid margins with flaky debris in the lashes. The conjunctiva is mildly and diffusely hyperemic	Recommend lid margin scrubs twice daily using cotton-tipped applicator with baby shampoo as initial therapy; warm compresses with heating pad or wet washrag for 10 min twice daily; short course of Tobradex if wash fails
Inflamed pinguecula	Fig. 5	Localized redness at the limbus, with mild-moderate ocular discomfort	Red mound in the nasal or temporal limbus	Prescribe OTC vasoconstrictors for 72 h; if not resolved, refer to ophthalmology
Pterygium	Fig. 6	Localized redness at the limbus with extension onto the cornea, with mild discomfort or no pain	Mounded triangular hyperemic area on the nasal or sometimes temporal conjunctiva pointing toward and extending onto the cornea	If interferes with visual field, then refer nonurgently to ophthalmology for excision

(continued on next page)

Table 1
(continued)

Condition	Appearance	Key Symptoms	Distinguishing Signs	Management
Subconjunctival hemorrhage	Fig. 7	Bright red area of conjunctiva without pain or change in vision	Blotchy redness confined to 1 area of conjunctiva	No treatment is necessary; if no history of coughing or straining, consider measuring blood pressure
Stye/hordeolum	Fig. 8	Pain, swelling, and redness of the lid	Focal inflammation of the lash follicle or its meibomian gland	Warm compresses
Corneal abrasion	Fig. 9	Red eye, pain, photophobia, typically with a history of trauma or foreign body	Markedly uncomfortable patient with tearing, photophobia, fluorescein staining of defect; ± presence of foreign body	Topical antibiotic therapy for 1 week; cycloplegics ± narcotics for pain relief. If abrasion caused by contact lens wear and opacifications are present in the cornea (suggestive of infectious keratitis), refer emergently to ophthalmology
Prompt (Within 1 d) or Nonurgent Referral to Ophthalmology				
Immunogenic conjunctivitis	Fig. 10	Minimal symptoms, other than mildly chronically red eye ± dryness	Mild, diffuse hyperemia of the conjunctiva without discharge	Refer chronically red eyes to ophthalmologist (nonurgently) for evaluation
Dacryocystitis	Fig. 11	Redness and swelling at inner corner of eye with pain/tenderness; in infants, associated with congenitally blocked nasolacrimal duct; in adults, associated with chronic sinusitis, trauma, or tumor	Redness of lacrimal sac and surrounding soft tissues, purulent discharge	Prompt referral to ophthalmologist for incision and draining along with broad-spectrum antibiotics
Cavernous sinus arteriovenous fistula	Fig. 12	Chronic red eye that may be painful	Conjunctival vessels with corkscrew appearance; sometimes with lid edema, proptosis, or ocular misalignment	Prompt referral to ophthalmology
Canaliculitis	Fig. 13	Chronic unilateral red eye, tearing, and discharge (watery or purulent)	Punctum orifice is swollen, red, and turned outward; tenderness with pericanalicular inflammation including surrounding conjunctivitis; discharge expressed with pressure on the punctum	Warm compresses, digital massage, topical antibiotic; prompt referral to ophthalmology for surgical management (canaliculotomy)

Orbital tumor	Fig. 14	Proptosis with or without pain and redness	Proptosis with variable hyperemia of conjunctiva; ± restricted extraocular movements, diplopia, ptosis or lid retraction	Order imaging to define the location and extent of the tumor; refer urgently to ophthalmology for management
Immediate Referral to Ophthalmology				
Anterior uveitis/iritis	Fig. 15	Periocular pain, photophobia with normal vision	Ciliary flush, ± irregular pupil	Refer immediately to ophthalmology
Episcleritis	Fig. 16	Ocular pain	Dilatation of conjunctival vessels in localized area remote from cornea, minimal discharge	Refer immediately to ophthalmology
Scleritis	Fig. 17	Ocular pain	Dilatation of conjunctival vessels in localized area remote from cornea, thinning of sclera in area over the site of inflammation (purple color of the underlying uvea shows through)	Refer immediately to ophthalmology
Keratitis	Fig. 18	Blurred vision, photophobia, periocular pain, foreign body sensation	Disrupted light reflex, ciliary flush, fluorescein staining of defect	Refer immediately to ophthalmology
Endophthalmitis	Fig. 19	Loss of vision, periocular pain	Diffusely red conjunctiva, swollen eyelids, hypopyon	Refer immediately to ophthalmology
Acute angle-closure glaucoma	Fig. 20	Severe ocular pain, photophobia, blurred vision	Ciliary flush, hazy cornea, nonreactive pupil (fixed, midposition)	Refer immediately to ophthalmology
Orbital cellulitis	Fig. 21	Periocular pain, swelling of upper and lower lids, diffuse conjunctival hyperemia	Tender eyelids and globes; distinguish whether the cellulitis is preseptal (anterior to the orbital septum) vs postseptal (extends behind the orbital septum) by determining whether extraocular movements are reduced and proptosis is present (which accompany postseptal orbital cellulitis)	Admission for treatment with IV antibiotics; sino-orbital imaging to define the extent of infection. Immediate ophthalmology consult

Abbreviations: IV, intravenous; NSAIDs, nonsteroidal antiinflammatory drugs; OTC, over the counter.
Data from Refs.[1–5,16]

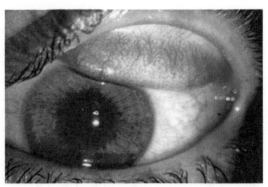

Fig. 1. Allergic conjunctivitis. (*From* La Rosa M, Lionetti E, Reibaldi M, et al. Allergic conjunctivitis: a comprehensive review of the literature. Ital J Pediatr 2013;39:18; with permission.)

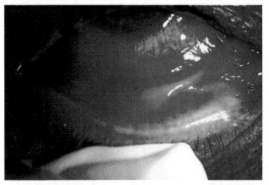

Fig. 2. Bacterial conjunctivitis. (*From* Baiyeroju A, Bowman R, Gilbert C, et al. Managing eye health in young children. Comm Eye Health 2010;23(72):10; with permission.)

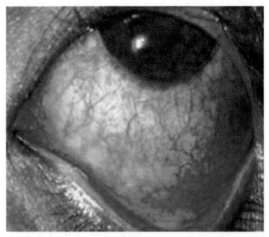

Fig. 3. Viral conjunctivitis. (*From* Lopez-Prats MJ, Marco ES, Hidalgo-Mora JJ, et al. Bleeding follicular conjunctivitis due to influenza H1N1 virus. J Ophthalmol 2010;2010:423672; with permission.)

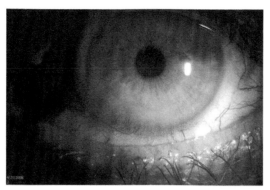

Fig. 4. Blepharitis. (*Courtesy of* Emory Eye Center, Emory University School of Medicine, Atlanta, GA; with permission.)

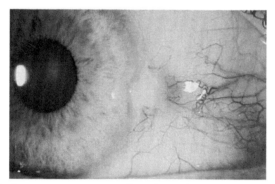

Fig. 5. Pinguecula. (*From* Ferri FF. Ferri's color atlas and text of clinical medicine. Philadelphia: Saunders Elsevier; 2009; with permission.)

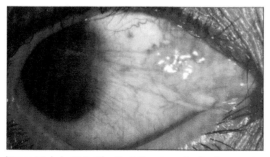

Fig. 6. Pterygium. (*From* Mahdy MA, Bhatia J. Treatment of primary pterygium: role of limbal stem cells and conjunctival autograft transplantation. Oman J Ophthalmol 2009;2:26; with permission.)

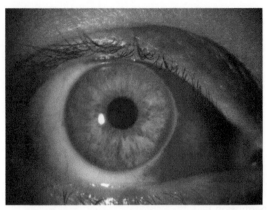

Fig. 7. Subconjunctival hemorrhage. (*From* Tarlan B, Kiratli H. Subconjunctival hemorrhage: risk factors and potential indicators. Clin Ophthalmol 2013;7:1165; with permission.)

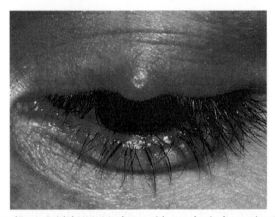

Fig. 8. Hordeolum. (*From* Seidel HM. Mosby's guide to physical examination. Philadelphia: Elsevier Mosby; 2003; with permission.)

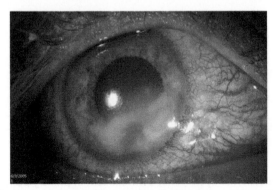

Fig. 9. Corneal abrasion. (*Courtesy of* Emory Eye Center, Emory University School of Medicine, Atlanta, GA; with permission.)

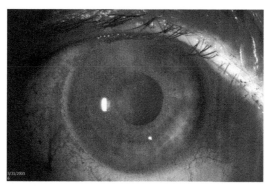

Fig. 10. Immunogenic conjunctivitis. (*Courtesy of* Emory Eye Center, Emory University School of Medicine, Atlanta, GA; with permission.)

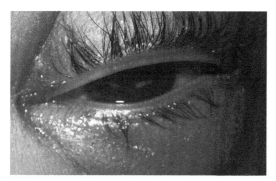

Fig. 11. Dacryocystitis. (*Courtesy of* Emory Eye Center, Emory University School of Medicine, Atlanta, GA; with permission.)

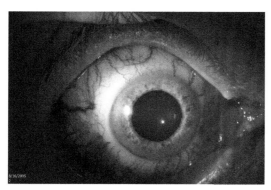

Fig. 12. Cavernous sinus arteriovenous fistula. (*Courtesy of* Emory Eye Center, Emory University School of Medicine, Atlanta, GA; with permission.)

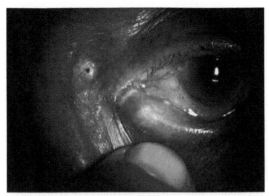

Fig. 13. Canaliculitis. (*From* Mohan ER, Kabra S, Udhay P, et al. Intracanalicular antibiotics may obviate the need for surgical management of chronic suppurative canaliculitis. Indian J Ophthalmol 2008;56(4):339; with permission.)

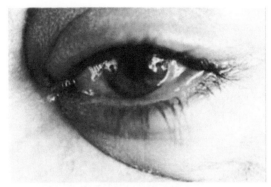

Fig. 14. Orbital tumor. (*From* Hassane S, Fouad E, Said I, et al. Orbital metastatic angiosarcoma. Korean J Ophthalmol 2010;24(6):364; with permission.)

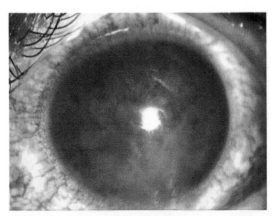

Fig. 15. Anterior uveitis. (*From* Takahashi YY, Kakizaki H, Ichionose AA, et al. Severe anterior uveitis associated with idiopathic dacryoadenitis in diabetes mellitus patient. Clin Ophthalmol 2011;5:620; with permission.)

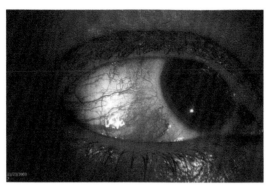

Fig. 16. Episcleritis. (*Courtesy of* Emory Eye Center, Emory University School of Medicine, Atlanta, GA; with permission.)

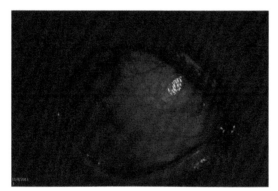

Fig. 17. Scleritis. (*Courtesy of* Emory Eye Center, Emory University School of Medicine, Atlanta, GA; with permission.)

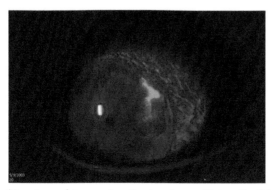

Fig. 18. Keratitis. (*Courtesy of* Emory Eye Center, Emory University School of Medicine, Atlanta, GA; with permission.)

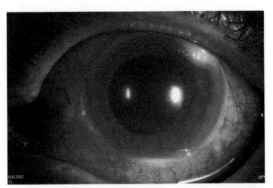

Fig. 19. Endophthalmitis with hypopyon. (*Courtesy of* Emory Eye Center, Emory University School of Medicine, Atlanta, GA; with permission.)

department equipped to handle more serious conditions and those that can be managed in the primary care setting. **Table 1** outlines the particular conditions that warrant immediate or prompt referral to an ophthalmologist along with those for which the primary care provider may initiate therapy.

If general, primary care providers may initiate therapy for conditions presenting with a red eye in which there is no foreign body sensation or photophobia, vision is unaffected, the pupil reacts, there is no hypopyon or hyphema, and there is no corneal opacity. In contrast, if any of the following red flags are present for a patient presenting with a red eye, even when the exact diagnosis is not known, the primary care provider should immediately refer to ophthalmology:

- Severe eye pain
- Loss of visual acuity or other visual deficits
- Loss of pupillary reactivity
- Unilateral red eye accompanied by discomfort and nausea, which is suggestive of acute angle-closure glaucoma
- Ulceration of the cornea as shown by a corneal infiltrate or opacity that stains with fluorescein examination

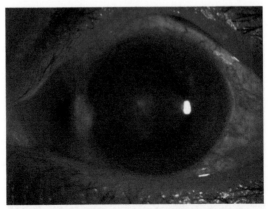

Fig. 20. Acute angle-closure glaucoma. (*From* Premsinthil M, Salowi MA, Siew CM, et al. Spontaneous malignant glaucoma in a patient with patent peripheral iridotomy. BMC Ophthalmol 2012;12:64; with permission.)

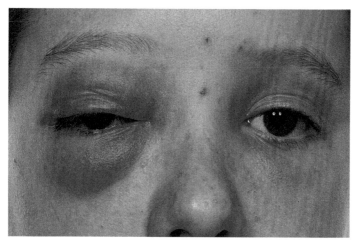

Fig. 21. Orbital cellulitis. (*From* Norris A, Rowe-Jones J. Infections and foreign bodies in the ear, nose and throat. Surgery 2006;24(9):301; with permission.)

- Hypopyon (a collection of white blood cells layering in the anterior chamber of the eye) or hyphema (a collection of red blood cells layering in the anterior chamber of the eye), suggestive of sight-threatening infection or trauma involving the eye.

REFERENCES

1. Wirbelauer C. Management of the red eye for the primary care physician. Am J Med 2006;119(4):302–6.
2. Leibowitz HM. The red eye. N Engl J Med 2000;343(5):345–51.
3. Cronau H, Kankanala RR, Mauger T. Diagnosis and management of red eye in primary care. Am Fam Physician 2010;81(2):137–44.
4. Peterson I, Hayward AC. Antibacterial prescribing in primary care. J Antimicro Chemoterh 2007;60(Suppl 1):i43–7.
5. Kunimoto DY, Kanitkar KD, Makar M. The Wills eye manual: office and emergency room diagnosis and treatment of eye disease. Philadelphia: Wolters Kluwer / Lippincott Williams & Wilkins; 2008.
6. Bahn RS. Graves' ophthalmopathy. N Engl J Med 2010;362:726.
7. Stern ME, Schaumburg CS, Pflugfelder SC. Dry eye as a mucosal autoimmune disease. Int Rev Immunol 2013;32:19.
8. Fujita M, Igarashi T, Kurai T, et al. Correlation between dry eye and rheumatoid arthritis activity. Am J Ophthalmol 2005;140:808.
9. Wu IB, Schwartz RA. Reiter's syndrome: the classic triad and more. J Am Acad Dermatol 2008;59:113.
10. Fessler BJ, Boumpas DT. Severe major organ involvement in systemic lupus erythematosus. Diagnosis and management. Rheum Dis Clin North Am 1995;21:81.
11. Harper SL, Letko E, Samson CM, et al. Wegener's granulomatosis: the relationship between ocular and systemic disease. J Rheumatol 2001;28:1025.
12. Kent PD, Michet CJ Jr, Luthra HS. Relapsing polychondritis. Curr Opin Rheumatol 2004;16:56.

13. Akova YA, Jabbur NS, Foster CS. Ocular presentation of polyarteritis nodosa: clinical course and management with steroid and cytotoxic therapy. Ophthalmology 1993;100(12):1775–81.
14. Jabs DA, Green WR, Fox R, et al. Ocular manifestations of acquired immune deficiency syndrome. Ophthalmology 1989;96(7):1092–9.
15. Newman-Casey PA, Talwar N, Nan B, et al. The relationship between components of metabolic syndrome and open-angle glaucoma. Ophthalmology 2011;118(7): 1318–26.
16. Patel SJ, Lundy DC. Ocular manifestations of autoimmune disease. Am Fam Physician 2002;66(6):991–8.

Herpes Zoster Ophthalmicus

Julie L. Johnson, MD*, Rianot Amzat, MD, MPH,
Nicolle Martin, MD, MPH

KEYWORDS

- Herpes zoster ophthalmicus • Shingles • HZO • Shingles complications
- Ophthalmic zoster

KEY POINTS

- Herpes zoster and herpes zoster ophthalmicus (HZO) are conditions that primary care practitioners will encounter in their careers. Early diagnosis and management are key elements to reducing some of the long-term sequelae of this condition.
- The main goals of management are to shorten the clinical course, to provide analgesia, and to prevent complications related to HZO.
- Ophthalmologic consultation is crucial if the diagnosis of HZO is a possibility. Inpatient management with intravenous antiviral therapy is preferred.
- The type of therapy provided is predicated on the area of ophthalmologic involvement.
- Vaccination with Zostavax significantly reduces the risk of developing shingles and zoster-related complications. It is advised to offer to those aged 60 years and older, but has been approved for use in 50 to 59 year olds.

BACKGROUND

Herpes zoster (HZ) is a commonly encountered disorder in primary care. It is caused by the human herpesvirus 3, the same virus that causes varicella (chickenpox) as the primary infection.[1] After the initial varicella infection, the virus may lay dormant in the neurosensory ganglia for years. Because of many factors (eg, age, stress, immunosuppression), there is reactivation of the previously dormant virus resulting in extraocular and ocular manifestations of HZ (shingles).[2–6]

Herpes zoster ophthalmicus (HZO) occurs when reactivation of the latent virus in the trigeminal ganglia involves the ophthalmic division of the nerve (**Fig. 1**). It represents approximately 10% to 20% of cases of HZ[7] with the frontal branch being most commonly involved. HZO may manifest with only the pain and rash characteristic of

Department of Family and Preventive Medicine, Emory University School of Medicine, 4500 North Shallowford Road, Suite B, Atlanta, GA 30338, USA
* Corresponding author.
E-mail address: julie.l.johnson@emory.edu

Prim Care Clin Office Pract 42 (2015) 285–303
http://dx.doi.org/10.1016/j.pop.2015.05.007
0095-4543/15/$ – see front matter © 2015 Elsevier Inc. All rights reserved.
primarycare.theclinics.com

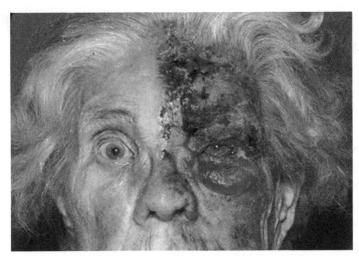

Fig. 1. Acute HZO. (*From* Groves N. Low use of herpes zoster vaccine raises concerns. Ophthalmology Times, 2014; with permission. Available at: http://ophthalmologytimes. modernmedicine.com/ophthalmologytimes/content/tags/clinical-diagnosis-ophthalmology/ low-use-herpes-zoster-vaccine-raise?page5full.)

HZ, without any involvement of ocular structures; however, it is estimated that 50% to 72% of patients experience direct ocular involvement.[8–15] Decreased cellular immunity has been found to play a role in increasing the risk of HZO. In HIV-infected patients, the risk of developing HZO has been reported to be 6.6 times higher than that of the general population.[7,16,17] Other risks factors include advancing age, use of immunosuppressive medications, and primary infection in infancy or in utero.[4,9,11,14,16,18–32]

PATHOPHYSIOLOGY

After the initial varicella infection, unless the immune system is compromised, the varicella zoster virus (VZV) usually stays dormant in the sensory ganglia or perineuronal cells. However, for reasons that are not fully understood, the virus reactivates from its dormant state in the sensory ganglion, starts to replicate, and then migrates peripherally along the sensory nerves, which triggers an immune response and inflammation of the connective tissue sheath surrounding each nerve (**Fig. 2**). This immune response and inflammation of the connective tissue sheath cause intense pain along the nerve distribution and locally result in skin blisters or ocular inflammation along the affected nerve distribution.[2–6]

SIGNS AND SYMPTOMS OF HERPES ZOSTER OPHTHALMICUS

HZO can present with either extraocular or ocular manifestations. In some cases, both symptom constellations can occur simultaneously. In the prodromal phase of HZO, patients usually complain of an influenza-like illness with fatigue, malaise, and low-grade fever. These symptoms may last up to 1 week before the eruption of a vesicular skin rash. Because the prodromal phase of HZO is similar to that of chickenpox, it is important to elicit a history of prior exposure. However, there are key features on the skin examination and on the eye examination that will distinguish the 2 conditions (**Table 1**).[9,11–14,18,21–25,27–31,33–35]

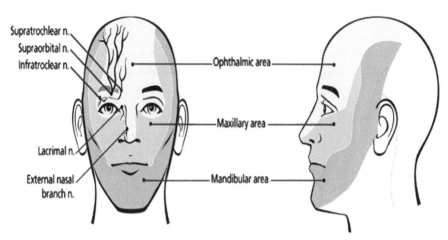

Fig. 2. Trigeminal nerve and dermatomes. (*From* Delengocky T, Bui CM. Complete ophthal-moplegia with pupillary involvement as an initial clinical presentation of herpes zoster oph-thalmicus. J Am Osteopath Assoc 2008;108:615–21; with permission.)

The rash of HZO usually starts on the forehead, accompanied by dermatomal pain in the distribution of the ophthalmic nerve. An erythematous papular rash develops in a dermatomal distribution, progressing into papules and vesicles that eventually erupt and then crust over.

A vesicular rash in the dermatome of the nasociliary nerve may indicate ophthalmic complications. Involvement of the tip of the nose (Hutchinson sign) is thought to be a predictor of ocular manifestations (**Fig. 3**). In some case series, 100% of patients with nasociliary involvement go on to develop ocular pathologic abnormality.[36]

CLINICAL MANIFESTATIONS

A wide range of symptoms affecting the eye may occur during the various phases of ophthalmic zoster.[4,8,9,11–14,18,21–25,27,29,30,33,35,37–44] Common symptoms may include eye pain, red eye, tearing, and decreased vision (**Table 2**).

Table 1 How to differentiate herpes zoster from varicella zoster (skin examination)		
	Chickenpox vs Shingles	
	Varicella Zoster Virus	**Herpes Zoster Virus**
Transmission	Through respiratory secretions, vesicular fluid	By reactivation of latent VZV
Signs and symptoms	Malaise, fever, rash	Neuralgia, dermatomal rash, weakness of affected nerve
Distribution of rash	Trunk initially; progressing to face, extremities, mucosa, or a combination	Primarily (50%) thoracic; remainder cranial, cervical lumber
Character of rash	Nongrouped, itchy vesicles	Grouped, markedly erythematous painful vesicles

Adapted from Brouwer RE. Shingles: a review of herpes zoster virus. Advance Healthcare Network, 1999. Available at: http://nurse-practitioners-and-physician-assistants.advanceweb.com/Article/Shingles-A-Review-of-Herpes-Zoster-Virus.aspx.

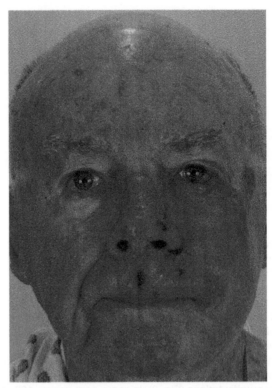

Fig. 3. Nasal involvement. (*From* Murrell GL, Hayes BH. Hutchinson sign and herpes zoster. Otolaryngol Head Neck Surg 2007;136(2):313–4; with permission.)

Table 2		
Symptoms of ophthalmic zoster		
Eye Structure	**Symptoms**	**Onset**
Eyelid	Macular rash in acute phase, which may progress to scarring, ptosis	With onset of rash
Conjuctiva	Swelling, injection, petechial hemorrhages	2–3 d, usually resolve within a week
Episclera/sclera	Diffuse or localized redness with dilatation of the deeper vessels, may lead to scleral atrophy in the chronic phase	1 wk
Cornea	Punctate epithelial keratitis, swollen corneal surface epithelial cells. In the chronic phase, there may be scarring, ulcers, and loss of corneal sensation	Variable depending on area of cornea from 4 days to months
Uvea	Uveitis[44]	2 weeks to years
Retina	Acute retinal necrosis	Varies
Cranial nerves	Optic neuritis, swollen, edematous optic nerve head, oculomotor palsies[38]	Varies

Data from Shaikh S, Ta CN. Evaluation and management of herpes zoster ophthalmicus. Am Fam Physician 2002;66(9):1723–30.

Blepharitis and Conjunctivitis

The eyelids and conjunctiva are commonly involved in HZO. Patients may present with ptosis due to edema. Conjunctivitis is one of the most common signs of acute HZO. The conjunctiva appears injected and edematous, often with petechial hemorrhages; these symptoms are commonly transient, lasting up to 1 week.

Episcleritis and Scleritis

The episclera and sclera may also be affected in HZO. Features include a localized or diffuse redness, associated with pain and swelling of the conjunctiva, and episclera.

Cornea

Corneal complications occur in approximately 65% of cases of HZO.[45] Corneal disease may be either superficial or interstitial and can result in significant visual loss. Patients present with decreased vision, light sensitivity, loss of cornea sensitivity, and pain. Features include punctate epithelial keratitis (earliest lesion noted in corneal involvement), dendritic keratitis (results in tree-branch-like epithelial defects), stromal keratitis, deep stromal keratitis, and neurotrophic keratopathy (erosions, persistent defects), which occur from months to years after infection (**Fig. 4**).[8,26,27,37,39,41,46]

EVALUATION

The physical examination in the patient with suspected HZO should include a comprehensive ophthalmologic examination, including external inspection, visual acuity assessment, detailed slit-lamp examination (including fluorescein and rose bengal staining), and posterior segment examination (**Fig. 5**). Diagnostic laboratory testing is rarely indicated, because diagnosis can usually be made by history and physical examination. If testing is necessary, a Tzanck smear or Wright stain can be used to determine whether lesions contain herpes-type virus. Viral culture, direct immunofluorescence assay, or polymerase chain reaction may also be used to confirm the diagnosis.[12,13,21,28,34,38,40,45,47]

DIFFERENTIAL DIAGNOSIS OF HERPES ZOSTER OPHTHALMICUS

The differential diagnosis of HZO includes a broad range of ocular pathologic abnormalities. Other viral infections such as herpes simplex may be confused with HZO (**Box 1, Table 3**). Herpes simplex may also cause a vesicular rash, but not typically dermatomal in distribution, and may cause a corneal ulcer, which is not usually seen in HZO. Other causes of corneal stromal inflammation include Epstein-Barr virus, mumps, and syphilis. Facial pain from HZO could originate from migraine headache, referred pain, and orbital tumors.[48]

MANAGEMENT OF HERPES ZOSTER OPHTHALMICUS

The goals of management in the patient with HZO are to shorten the clinical course, to provide analgesia and to prevent potential complications.[2,3,5,6,12,13,15,20,28,33,40,42,43,45,46,49–64] According to the Centers for Disease Control and Prevention (CDC) Advisory Committee on Immunization Practices (ACIP), approximately 1 in 3 persons will develop zoster during their lifetime, resulting in an estimated 1 million episodes in the United States annually (**Fig. 6**). The risk for postherpetic neuralgia (PHN) in patients with zoster is 10% to 18%. The second most common complication of zoster is eye involvement, which occurs in 10% to 25% of zoster

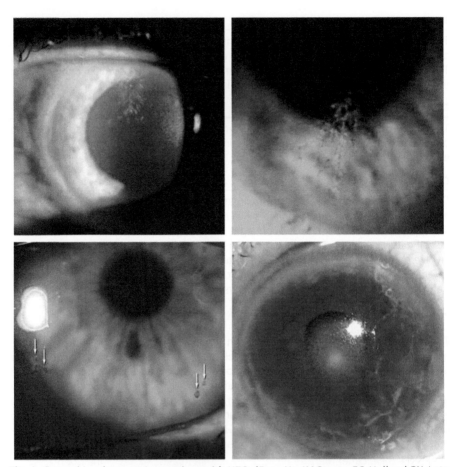

Fig. 4. Corneal involvement in a patient with HZO. (*From* Hu AY, Strauss EC, Holland GN. Late varicella-zoster virus dendriform keratitis in patients with histories of herpes zoster ophthalmicus. Am J Ophthalmol 2010;149(2):214–220; with permission.)

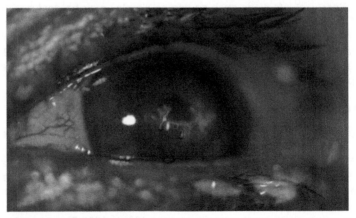

Fig. 5. Dendrites observed under fluorescein. (*From* Catron T, Hern HG. Herpes zoster ophthalmicus. West J Emerg Med 2008;9(3):174–6.)

Box 1
Differential diagnosis of herpes zoster ophthalmicus

Conditions causing similar external appearance
- Herpes simplex
- Ulcerative blepharitis

Conditions causing corneal stromal inflammation
- Epstein-Barr virus
- Mumps
- Syphilis

Conditions causing associated facial pain
- Migraine headache
- Orbital pseudotumor
- Orbital cellulitis
- Referred pain from toothache

episodes and can result in prolonged or permanent pain, facial scarring, and loss of vision. Approximately 3% of patients with zoster are hospitalized; many of these episodes involved persons with one or more immunocompromising conditions. Deaths attributable to zoster are uncommon among persons who are not immunocompromised.[56,65]

In terms of the frequency of types of ophthalmic complications associated with HZ, keratitis (76%) was the overwhelming form of presentation based on population-based original research conducted by researchers at the Mayo Clinic.[66,67] Keratitis was followed by uveitis/iritis (46.6%), conjunctivitis (35.4%), severe eye pain (14%), increased intraocular pressure (13.2%), scleritis/episcleritis (10.6%), and corneal scarring (10%). Other manifestations occurred in less than 10% of the population.[8,66]

Based on their medical record review, Yawn and colleagues[66] discovered that recurrent keratitis and recurrent iritis/uveitis occurred in 6.9% and 7.4%, respectively. Outcomes included 6 (3.3%) patients with new vision decrements to 20/200 or worse. Two individuals had successful corneal transplants. Another 6 (3.3%) individuals had

Table 3		
How to differentiate herpes simplex from varicella zoster		
Feature	**Herpes Simplex**	**Varicella Zoster**
Epithelium	Linear defect with bare stroma that is surrounded by edematous epithelial cells	Elevated, painted-on appearance
Staining	Ulcer base stains with fluorescein; diseased borders of epithelial cells stain with rose bengal	Minimal fluorescein staining
Terminal bulbs	Frequent	None

Similarly to herpes simplex virus keratitis, an active varicella zoster infection of the epithelium subsequently may invade neighboring epithelial cells.

Adapted from Marcolini W. Varicella zoster virus: from chickenpox to shingles. Review of Optometry. 2013. Available at: http://www.reviewofoptometry.com/continuing_education/tabviewtest/lessonid/108881.

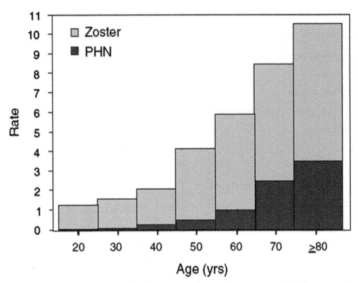

Fig. 6. Rate (per 1000 person-years) of zoster and PHN by age: United States. (*From* Harpaz R, Ortega-Sanchez IR, Seward JF, Advisory Committee on Immunization Practices (ACIP) Centers for Disease Control and Prevention (CDC). Prevention of herpes zoster: recommendations of the Advisory Committee on Immunization Practices (ACIP). MMWR Recomm Rep 2008;57:1–30.)

lid ptosis that affected vision, including one elderly woman with a permanent unilateral tarsorrhaphy. Severe HZ eye pain was reported to be directly responsible for one unsuccessful suicide attempt.

The annual medical care cost of treating incident HZ cases in the United States, extrapolated from the results of one population-based study, is estimated at $1.1 billion. Most of the costs are for the care of immunocompetent adults with HZ, especially among those 50 years and older.[67]

PREVENTION

An ounce of prevention is worth a pound of cure
—Benjamin Franklin

In 1995, the US Food and Drug Administration (FDA) licensed a live-attenuated varicella vaccine for immunization of healthy infants, children, adolescents, and adults in the United States who have not had chickenpox and who are not pregnant. Studies have shown that the varicella vaccine in children is highly effective in preventing chickenpox. Nevertheless, reports exist of outbreaks of varicella disease in highly immunized groups. Therefore, changes to the current vaccination policy may be anticipated.[15,53,56,65]

Based on the results of the Shingles Prevention Study, in 2006, the FDA approved the Zostavax vaccine for the prevention of HZ in people aged 60 years and older. More than 38,000 adults older than 60 years were enrolled in a randomized, double-blind, placebo-controlled trial of the vaccine. The vaccine reduced the incidence of HZ by 61.1% and the incidence of PHN by 66.5%.[15,53,56,65]

In March 2011, the FDA lowered the approved age for use of Zostavax to 50 to 59 years. Zostavax was already approved for use in individuals aged 60 years or older.

Annually, in the United States, shingles affects approximately 200,000 healthy people aged 50 to 59 years. Approval was based on a multicenter study, the Zostavax Efficacy and Safety Trial.[56] The trial was conducted in the United States and 4 other countries in 22,439 people aged 50 to 59 years. Participants were randomized in a 1:1 ratio to receive either Zostavax or placebo. Participants were monitored for at least 1 year to see if shingles developed. Compared with placebo, Zostavax significantly reduced the risk of developing zoster by approximately 70%.[15,53,56,65]

The burden of HZ increases as a person ages, with steep increases occurring after age 50 years. Not only does the risk of HZ itself increase with age, but also among persons who experience HZ, older persons are much more likely to experience PHN, non-pain complications, hospitalizations, and interference with activities of daily living **(Table 4)**.[4,7,9,37,49,67–74] Because persons aged 50 years can expect to live an additional 32 years and persons aged 60 years, another 23 years, vaccination must offer durable effectiveness to protect against this increasing burden of disease.[53,56,65]

At the October 2013 meeting, the ACIP reviewed results from an updated cost-effectiveness analysis comparing health outcomes, health care resource utilization, costs, and quality-adjusted life years (QALYs) related to HZ, PHN, and nonpain complications among unvaccinated persons and persons vaccinated at either age 50, 60, or 70 years.[4,7,9,37,49,53,56,65,66,68–74]

Based on their projection of outcomes in persons aged 50 to 99 years, vaccination at age 60 years would prevent the most shingles cases (26,147 cases per 1 million persons) followed by vaccination at age 70 years, and then age 50 years (preventing 21,269 and 19,795 cases, respectively). However, vaccination at age 70 years would prevent the most cases of PHN (6439 cases per 1 million persons), followed by age 60 years, and then age 50 years (preventing 2698 and 941 PHN cases, respectively). From a societal perspective, vaccinating at age 70, 60, and 50 years would cost $37,000, $86,000, and $287,000 per QALY saved, respectively.[4,7,9,37,49,66,68–74] The high cost per QALY saved with vaccination at age 50 years results from limited impact on prevention of PHN and other complications from ages 50 through 59 years and no remaining vaccine protection after age 60 when risk for PHN and other complications increases sharply.[4,7,9,37,49,53,56,65,66,68–74]

Table 4
Impact of acute herpes zoster and postherpetic neuralgia on quality of life

Life Factor	Impact
Physical	Chronic fatigue
	Anorexia and weight loss
	Physical inactivity
	Insomnia
Psychological	Anxiety
	Difficulty concentrating
	Depression, suicidal ideation
Social	Fewer social gatherings
	Changes in social role
Functional	Interferes with activities of daily living (eg, dressing, bathing, eating, travel, cooking, and shopping)

From Harpaz R, Ortega-Sanchez IR, Seward JF, Advisory Committee on Immunization Practices (ACIP) Centers for Disease Control and Prevention (CDC). Prevention of herpes zoster: recommendations of the Advisory Committee on Immunization Practices (ACIP). MMWR Recomm Rep 2008;57:1–30.

Considering that the burden of HZ and its complications increases with age and that the duration of vaccine protection in persons aged 60 years and older is uncertain, the ACIP maintained its current recommendation that HZ vaccine be routinely recommended for adults aged 60 years and older (**Fig. 7**).[15,53,56,65] Despite all of its benefits, the vaccination is not without risks and should be used with caution in certain populations (**Table 5**).[15]

Other methods of prevention of initial infection include contact and respiratory isolation of infected patients until full crusting of lesions is achieved as well as postexposure prophylaxis with varicella zoster immune globulin (VZIG) in select populations.[25,35,39,57–60,75,76]

IMMUNOLOGIC THERAPY

The CDC recommends administration of VZIG to prevent or modify clinical illness in persons with exposure to varicella or HZ who are susceptible or immunocompromised. It should be reserved for patients at risk for severe disease and complications, such as neonates and patients who are immunocompromised or pregnant.[25,35,39,57–60] VZIG provides maximum benefit when administered as soon as possible after the presumed exposure, but it may be effective if administered as late as 96 hours after exposure. Protection after VZIG administration lasts for an average of approximately 3 weeks, according to the CDC.[25,35,39,57–60]

PHARMACOLOGIC ANTIVIRAL TREATMENT

Oral acyclovir (5 times per day) has been shown to shorten the duration of signs and symptoms as well as to reduce the incidence and severity of HZO complications. Although it can reduce the pain during the acute phase, it has no demonstrated effect on reducing the incidence or severity of PHN.[25,35,39,57–60] Acyclovir appears to benefit patients the most when therapy is initiated within 72 hours of onset of the skin lesions,

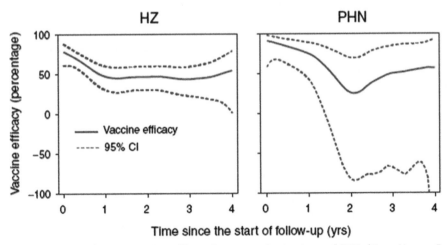

Fig. 7. Duration of zoster vaccine efficacy for preventing zoster and PHN. (*From* Harpaz R, Ortega-Sanchez IR, Seward JF, Advisory Committee on Immunization Practices (ACIP) Centers for Disease Control and Prevention (CDC). Prevention of herpes zoster: recommendations of the Advisory Committee on Immunization Practices (ACIP). MMWR Recomm Rep 2008;57:1–30.)

Table 5	
Herpes zoster ophthalmicus vaccine contraindications	
Herpes Zoster Vaccine Contraindicated	**Herpes Zoster Vaccine Not Contraindicated**
Leukemia or lymphoma or other malignancies of the bone marrow or lymphatic system	Patients with cancer in remission and off chemotherapy and radiation for ≥3 mo
AIDS/HIV with CD+4 ≤200 mm^3 or ≤15% total lymphocytes	Topical corticosteroids
≥20 mg/d prednisone for ≥14 d, or other immunosuppressive medications	Corticosteroid injections into joint/bursa/tendon
Use of >0.4 mg/kg/wk methotrexate, or >3 mg/kg/d azathioprine, or >1.5 mg/kg/d mercaptopurine	Inhaled corticosteroids
Pregnancy	<20 mg/d prednisone or <14 d of corticosteroids
Active, untreated tuberculosis	≤0.4 mg/kg/wk methotrexate
Hematopoietic stem cell transplantation <24 mo	≤3 mg/kg/d azathioprine
Treatment with adalimumab (Humira, Abbott Laboratories), infliximab (Remicade, Centocor Ortho Biotech), or etanercept (Enbrel; Amgen, Pfizer)	≤1.5 mg/kg/d mercaptopurine

Adapted from Lohr LK. Prevention, treatment of herpes zoster pose challenges for patients with cancer. Infectious Disease News. September 2013.

with higher complication rates occurring among patients whose treatment was delayed.[25,35,39,57–60]

Both famciclovir (500 mg 3 times a day) and valacyclovir (1 g 3 times a day) have been shown to be as effective as acyclovir (800 mg 5 times a day) in the treatment of HZ and reduction in complications.[25,35,39,57–60] Like acyclovir, these agents are approved in the United States for the management of HZ. These medications have simpler dosing regimens than acyclovir, which may increase patient compliance.[25,35,39,57–60]

A once-daily regimen of famciclovir 750 mg has been shown to reduce the cutaneous symptoms and pain of HZ as effectively as the standard regimen.[25,35,39,57–60] Although this simpler regimen might enhance compliance, it may not have any effect on ocular disease or postherpetic neuralgia.[25,35,39,57–60]

The effectiveness of antiviral therapy started more than 72 hours after symptom onset is not clearly established, and there is no evidence against the benefits of antiviral agents even after 72 hours. Theoretically, the ongoing viral replication can be deterred at any time if the rash continues, especially if new lesions appear.[25,35,39,57–60]

The standard duration of antiviral therapy for HZ is 7 to 10 days. Nevertheless, VZV DNA has been shown to persist in the cornea for up to 30 days; this is especially true in elderly individuals. This finding implies that the antiviral regimens may have to be continued, particularly for immunocompromised and elderly patients, although no clinical trials have proven their efficacy in this particular patient population. More serious complications, such as retinal involvement, may require days of intravenous (IV) therapy and months of oral antiviral therapy.[25,35,39,57–60]

Table 6 summarizes the indication, dose, and duration of each antiviral that can be used to treat this condition.[2,3,6,12,13,49,51,57,58,60,62,63]

Table 6
Treatments for varicella, shingles, and complications

Drug and Dose	Duration
Progressive outer retinal necrosis	
Ganciclovir: 5 mg/kg IV q12h +	Consult with expert
Foscarnet: 90 mg/kg IV q12h +	
Optimize antiretroviral therapy +	
Intravitreal Ganciclovir: 2.0 mg/0.05 mL twice/week and/or	
Intravitreal Foscarnet: 1.2 mg/0.05 mL twice weekly	
Acute retinal necrosis	
Acyclovir: 10 mg/kg IV q8h × 10–14 d followed by	8 wk total
Valacyclovir: 1000 mg PO tid × 6 wk	
HZ: acute localized dermatomal zoster (shingles)	
Valacyclovir: 1000 mg PO tid	7–10 d (longer if
Famciclovir: 500 mg PO tid	slow to resolve)
Acyclovir: 800 mg PO 5×/d	
HZ: extensive cutaneous lesions or visceral involvement	
Acyclovir: 10–15 mg/kg IV q8h until clinical improvement is evident, then switch to oral therapy as listed above for acute localized dermatomal zoster to complete 10–14-d course	10–14 d
Acyclovir-resistant VZV	
Foscarnet: 90 mg/kg IV q12h	14–28 d
Varicella (chickenpox): uncomplicated cases	
Acyclovir: 800 mg PO 5×/d	5–7 d
Valacyclovir: 1000 mg PO tid	
Famciclovir: 500 mg PO tid	
Varicella (chickenpox): severe or complicated cases	
Acyclovir: 10–15 mg/kg IV q8h; may switch to oral acyclovir, famciclovir, or valacyclovir (as dosed above for uncomplicated cases) if no evidence of visceral involvement	7–10 d
Foscarnet: 90 mg/kg IV q12h	14–28 d

Abbreviations: PO, orally; q8h, every 8 hours; q12h, every 12 hours; tid, 3 times a day.
Adapted from Casper C. Dermatologic manifestations. HIV web study: case based modules. University of Washington. Available at: http://depts.washington.edu/hivaids/derm/case4/discussion.html.

CORTICOSTEROID THERAPY

The use of oral corticosteroids reduces the duration of pain during the acute phase of the disease and increases the rate of cutaneous healing. However, it has not been shown to decrease the incidence of PHN.[23,25,35,39,57–60] Although steroids do improve quality of life, they are not appropriate for all patients and should be reserved for those patients who are relatively healthy and in whom there is no contraindication.[25,35,39,57–60]

Corticosteroids are recommended for HZO only for use in combination with antiviral agents. Corticosteroid therapy should not be used in patients at risk for corticosteroid-induced toxicity (eg, diabetes mellitus or gastritis).

Topical steroids alone do not reactivate the virus but may exacerbate spontaneous recurrences. In addition, although steroid eye drops may be beneficial for HZO, they are helpful only in certain ocular diseases (see later discussion) and can exacerbate others (ie, epithelial keratitis). Therefore, ophthalmologic consultation is mandatory before initiating ocular steroid therapy.[25,35,39,57–60]

ANESTHETICS, ANTIDEPRESSANTS, ANTICONVULSANTS, AND OTHER ADJUVANT THERAPY

Consideration of PHN should occur if a patient complains of severe pain at any point at or beyond the appearance of crusted vesicles. Treatment of PHN is complex. A multi-faceted, patient-specific approach is important.[25,35,39,57–60]

Clinical trials have shown that opioids, tricyclic antidepressants, and anticonvulsants (carbamazepine, gabapentin) may reduce the severity or duration of PHN, either as single agents or in combination. Topical application of lidocaine patches or capsaicin cream may provide relief for some patients. Consultation with a pain therapist may be required.[25,35,39,57–60]

Pavan-Langston has outlined the following protocol for treatment of PHN, which was supported by other reviews[10,25,27–30,35,39–41,53,57–60,64]:

- Tricyclic antidepressants: nortriptyline, amitriptyline, or desipramine 25 mg; adjust up to 75 mg at bedtime (every night at bedtime); for several weeks if needed
- Topical treatment with capsaicin ointment daily or 4 times per day or lidocaine patches
- Gabapentin (Neurontin, 30–600 mg 3 times a day) or sustained-release oxycodone (OxyContin SR, 10–20 mg 2 times a day).[25,35,39,57–60]

In one study, administration of lidocaine 4% ophthalmic eye drops produced a significant reduction in eye and forehead pain. Analgesic onset was noted within 15 minutes after administration and persisted for a median of 36 hours.[25,35,39,57–60]

Although anesthesia-based interventions such as local anesthetic blocking of sympathetic nerves or stellate ganglion blockade may produce transient relief, their effectiveness in reducing the protracted pain is still in question. Transcutaneous electric nerve stimulation and, if necessary, neurosurgery (eg, thermocoagulation of substantia gelatinosa rolandi) have been found to be helpful in exceptional cases.[13,25,35,39,49,53,54,57–60]

NONPHARMACOLOGIC STRATEGIES (SURGICAL)

Nonpharmacologic therapies that may be considered for acute zoster-associated pain include sympathetic, intrathecal, and epidural nerve blocks and percutaneous electrical nerve stimulation.[13,49,53,54,59] Although well-controlled studies are few, meta-analyses and clinical trials suggest that these treatments are effective in treating acute zoster-associated pain.[19,25,35,39,53,57–60] Rhizotomy (surgical separation of pain fibers) may be considered in cases of extreme, intractable pain.[19,25,35,39,57–60]

Some patients may require minor surgical procedures to correct scarring, such as a lateral tarsorrhaphy or lid traction sutures. In other patients with widespread corneal scarring, penetrating keratoplasty may be performed.[19,25,35,39,57–60,69]

REFERRAL STRATEGIES, CONSULTATIONS, AND COMANAGEMENT

Each specific ophthalmic complication due to HZO has specific treatment modalities, and these should be initiated in consultation with an ophthalmologist (**Table 7**).[19,25,35,39,43,45,49,50,57–60] The following is the recommended treatment by Shaikh and Ta in their review of HZO.[45]

- Blepharitis/conjunctivitis: Palliative, with cool compresses and topical lubrication; topical antibiotics for secondary infections
- Stromal keratitis: Topical steroids

Table 7
Chronic problems of acute herpes zoster ophthalmicus

Acute Herpes Zoster Ophthalmicus		Chronic Problems	
No ocular involvement Mild pain	Warm compresses	Anterior segment	Lateral tarsorrhaphy Transplant
Dendritic keratitis	Topical debridement Topical antibiotics	Chronic postherpetic neuralgia	Tricyclic antidepressants Terphenazme Capsaicin cream Gabapentin
Disciform disease iritis	Topical corticosteroids Cycloplegia	Lancinating pain	Carbamazepine
Immunocompetent individuals	Acyclovir 800 mg PO 5 times daily for 10 d	Uncontrolled pain	Sympathetic blockade Trigeminal ganglion ablation Valacyclovir 1 g 3 times daily for 7–14 d
Immunocompromised individuals	Acyclovir IV 10 mg/kg every 8 h for 7 d	Not applicable	Not applicable
Pain	Nonnarcotic or narcotic analgesia Cimetidine Artificial tears	Not applicable	Not applicable
Pain in immunocompetent individuals only	Prednisone 20 mg PO 3 times daily, then taper in 14 d[a]	—	—
Cerebral vasculitis	Acyclovir IV Corticosteroids IV	Not applicable	Not applicable

[a] Not an FDA-approved indication.
Courtesy of Comprehensive Ophthalmology Update, LLC; with permission.

- Neurotrophic keratitis: Topical lubrication; topical antibiotics for secondary infections; tissue adhesives and protective contact lenses to prevent corneal perforation
- Uveitis: Topical steroids; oral steroids; oral acyclovir; cycloplegics
- Scleritis/episcleritis: Topical nonsteroidal anti-inflammatory agents and steroids
- Acute retinal necrosis/progressive outer retinal necrosis: IV acyclovir (1500 mg per m² per day divided into 3 doses) for 7 to 10 days, followed by oral acyclovir (800 mg orally 5 times daily) for 14 weeks; laser/surgical intervention

The following consultations may be indicated[19,25,35,39,57–60]:

- Ophthalmologic consultation is crucial if the diagnosis of HZO is a possibility.
- Anesthesia consultation may be helpful for patients with refractory pain.
- Surgical consultation is occasionally required for debridement of involved epithelium.
- Psychiatric consultation may be necessary in patients with excruciating pain due to PHN, and severe depression related to the condition.
- An infectious disease specialist should be considered in cases of disseminated zoster or zoster with visceral involvement.

SELF-MANAGEMENT STRATEGIES

One of the most important things patients can do for themselves is prevention (via vaccination). As health care provides, taking every opportunity during each patient encounter to educate them regarding the benefits of the vaccine, will ward off the complications of the disease, for those patients aged 50 years and older. However, it is important to advise patients regarding their insurances covering the vaccination before age 60.

Because this complication occurs mostly in immunocompromised patients, compliance with HIV medication therapy is strongly encouraged as well as with diabetic glucose control.

There are no specific dietary recommendations in the patient with HZO except for adhering to the diet recommended based on their chronic conditions (diabetes, chronic kidney disease, and so on).

Patients with shingles can perform activities as tolerated. Most are capable of self-restricting their activities on the basis of any limitations that may be imposed by pain; additional advice from physicians is rarely, if ever, necessary.[19]

During the acute phase of the infection, patients should be counseled to avoid direct skin contact with immunocompromised persons, pregnant women, and individuals with no history of chickenpox infection. If the patient is hospitalized, contact isolation measures should be considered.[19,75,76]

Skin care can be achieved at home with simple instructions. Wet-to-dry dressings with sterile saline solution or Burow's solution (pharmacologic preparation made of 5% aluminum acetate dissolved in water) should be applied to the affected skin for 30 to 60 minutes 4 to 6 times per day.[25,35,39,57–60]

Calamine lotion, a mixture of zinc oxide with about 0.5% iron (III) oxide, may be used as an antipruritic (anti-itching) agent. It is also used as a mild antiseptic to prevent infections that can be caused by scratching the affected area as well as an astringent for weeping or oozing blisters. There is no evidence that calamine lotion has any real therapeutic effect on rashes and itching.[25,35,39,57–60]

DEVELOPING TREATMENTS

According to Sanjay and colleagues,[42] the herpes virus causes inflammatory destruction of the nerves, resulting in corneal hypoesthesia; this eventually causes neuropathic keratopathy. Researchers have been engaged in studies to revitalize sensitivity to the cornea.[42] Substance P and its derivatives are vital components in corneal sensation. In animal trials, these derivatives have been shown to stimulate corneal epithelial migration in vitro and corneal epithelial wound closure in vivo.[42] Based on their findings, eye drops containing tetrapeptides derived from substance P and insulin-like growth factor-1 showed successful epithelialization of defects in 73% of the study group within 4 weeks, resulting in regeneration of corneal nerve fibers.[42]

In another small case series study, the use of sterile eye drops containing thymosin β4 was reported to produce dramatic healing of geographic defects in 66% of the study group.[42,52] Ocular irritation was reduced in 100% of patients after the initiation of treatment.[42]

Finally, use of the Boston keratoprosthesis ("artificial cornea") is an option that has salvaged and restored vision in one case report of a patient with a severely damaged cornea secondary to HZO.[42] In this case report, the procedure was considered only after all conventional therapies had failed, and conventional keratoplasty was deemed highly unlikely to succeed.[42]

Amniotic membrane use is another intervention with some success.[43,61] Common uses for amniotic membrane for the ocular surface include nonhealing epithelial defects for conditions such as herpes simplex, zoster keratitis, and other conditions. The tissue can also be used after superficial keratectomy as an adjunctive therapy to assist with pain control and enhance epithelial healing.

The use of amniotic membrane and devices including Prokera (BIOTiSSUE) or Ambiodisk with Kontur lens (IOP Ophthalmics) is now approved by most insurance companies.[43,61]

SUMMARY

In US population studies, an estimated 1 million cases of HZ develop annually. According to the CDC, almost 1 of 3 people in the United States will develop shingles during their lifetime. Consequently, primary care providers are on the front lines of recognizing and managing the condition when it presents. Expeditious treatment will help minimize the complications and long-term sequelae of the disease.

Approximately 1% to 4% of people who get shingles are hospitalized for complications. HZO is the one of the most common complications, second only to PHN. HZO is preferably managed in the hospital setting with IV antivirals and in consultation with an ophthalmologist. HZO can involve various portions of the eye, and the area of involvement will dictate the type of treatment required. Other treatment options include anticonvulsants, opioid and non-opioid analgesics, antidepressants, and other adjuvant therapy to manage the pain.

Enlisting the collaboration of other specialists (eg, pain management, infectious diseases) may also be required to aid in the management of some of the complications. However, primary prevention using the Zostavax vaccine is the most cost-effective measure to thwart the disease and the long-term outcomes.

REFERENCES

1. Insinga RP, Itzler RF, Pellissier JM, et al. The incidence of herpes zoster in a United States administrative database. J Gen Intern Med 2005;20:748–53.
2. Harding SP. Management of ophthalmic zoster. J Med Virol 1993;(Suppl 1): 97–101.
3. Harding SP. Oral acyclovir in herpes zoster ophthalmicus. Eye (Lond) 1995;9(Pt 3):390–2.
4. Harding SP, Lipton JR, Wells JC. Natural history of herpes zoster ophthalmicus: predictors of postherpetic neuralgia and ocular involvement. Br J Ophthalmol 1987;71(5):353–8.
5. Harding SP, Lipton JR, Wells JC, et al. Relief of acute pain in herpes zoster ophthalmicus by stellate ganglion block. Br Med J (Clin Res Ed) 1986;292(6533):1428.
6. Harding SP, Porter SM. Oral acyclovir in herpes zoster ophthalmicus. Curr Eye Res 1991;10(Suppl):177–82.
7. Ragozzino MW, Melton LJ 3rd, Kurland LT, et al. Population-based study of herpes zoster and its sequelae. Medicine (Baltimore) 1982;61(5):310–6.
8. Liesegang TJ. Corneal complications from herpes zoster ophthalmicus. Ophthalmology 1985;92(3):316–24.
9. Liesegang TJ. Herpes zoster ophthalmicus natural history, risk factors, clinical presentation, and morbidity. Ophthalmology 2008;115(2 Suppl):S3–12.
10. Pavan-Langston D. Viral diseases of the ocular anterior segment. In: Foster C, Azar D, Dohlman C, editors. Smolin and Thofts. The Cornea. Scientific

foundations and clinical practice. 4th edition. Philadephia: Lippincott Williams and Wilkins; 2005. p. 297–397.

11. Liesegang TJ. Herpes zoster ophthalmicus. Int Ophthalmol Clin 1985;25(1): 77–96.

12. Liesegang TJ. Ophthalmic herpes zoster: diagnosis and antiviral therapy. Geriatrics 1991;46(10):64–6, 69–71.

13. Liesegang TJ. Diagnosis and therapy of herpes zoster ophthalmicus. Ophthalmology 1991;98(8):1216–29.

14. Liesegang TJ. Varicella-zoster virus eye disease. Cornea 1999;18(5):511–31.

15. Liesegang TJ. Varicella zoster virus vaccines: effective, but concerns linger. Can J Ophthalmol 2009;44(4):379–84.

16. Sandor EV, Millman A, Croxson TS, et al. Herpes zoster ophthalmicus in patients at risk for the acquired immune deficiency syndrome (AIDS). Am J Ophthalmol 1986;101(2):153–5.

17. Hodge WG, Seiff SR, Margolis TP. Ocular opportunistic infection incidences among patients who are HIV positive compared to patients who are HIV negative. Ophthalmology 1998;105:895–900.

18. Ang LP, Au Eong KG, Ong SG. Herpes zoster ophthalmicus. J Pediatr Ophthalmol Strabismus 2001;38(3):174–6.

19. Papadopoulos AJ, Birnkrant AP, Schwartz RA, et al. Childhood herpes zoster. Cutis 2001;68(1):21–3.

20. Revere K, Davidson SL. Update on management of herpes keratitis in children. Curr Opin Ophthalmol 2013;24(4):343–7.

21. Catron T, Hern HG. Herpes zoster ophthalmicus. West J Emerg Med 2008;9(3): 174–6.

22. Cockburn DM, Douglas IS. Herpes zoster ophthalmicus. Clin Exp Optom 2000; 83(2):59–64.

23. Dawodu OA, Osahon AI, Alikah AA, et al. Herpes zoster ophthalmicus. S Afr Med J 2005;95(1):30–1.

24. Gurwood AS, Savochka J, Sirgany BJ. Herpes zoster ophthalmicus. Optometry 2002;73(5):295–302.

25. Marsh RJ, Cooper M. Ophthalmic herpes zoster. Eye (Lond) 1993;7(Pt 3):350–70.

26. Omoti AE, Omoti CE. Maxillary herpes zoster with corneal involvement in a HIV positive pregnant woman. Afr J Reprod Health 2007;11(1):133–6.

27. Pavan-Langston D. Varicella-zoster ophthalmicus. Int Ophthalmol Clin 1975; 15(4):171–85.

28. Pavan-Langston D. Diagnosis and therapy of common eye infections: bacterial, viral, fungal. Compr Ther 1983;9(5):33–42.

29. Pavan-Langston D. Herpes zoster ophthalmicus. Neurology 1995;45(12 Suppl 8): S50–1.

30. Pavan-Langston D, Dunkel EC. Herpes zoster ophthalmicus. Compr Ther 1989; 15(5):3–9.

31. Stawell RJ, Hall AJ. Eye signs in systemic disease. Aust Fam Physician 2002; 31(3):217–23.

32. Thomas SL, Hall AJ. What does epidemiology tell us about risk factors for herpes zoster? Lancet Infect Dis 2004;4(1):26–33.

33. Edell AR, Cohen EJ. Herpes simplex and herpes zoster eye disease: presentation and management at a city hospital for the underserved in the United States. Eye Contact Lens 2013;39(4):311–4.

34. Opstelten W, Zaal MJ. Diagnostic tips for ophthalmic zoster. J Fam Pract 2008; 57(2):81.

35. Ritterband DC, Friedberg DN. Virus infections of the eye. Rev Med Virol 1998; 8(4):187–201.
36. Zaal MJ, Volker-Dieben HJ, D'Amaro J. Prognostic value of Hutchinson's sign in acute herpes zoster ophthalmicus. Graefes Arch Clin Exp Ophthalmol 2003; 241(3):187–91.
37. Camuglia JE, Beltz JE, Khurana K, et al. An unusual cause of visual loss after Herpes zoster ophthalmicus: a case report. Cases J 2010;3(1):17.
38. Jude E, Chakraborty A. Images in clinical medicine. Left sixth cranial nerve palsy with herpes zoster ophthalmicus. N Engl J Med 2005;353(16):e14.
39. Marsh RJ, Cooper M. Ophthalmic zoster: mucous plaque keratitis. Br J Ophthalmol 1987;71(10):725–8.
40. Pavan-Langston D. Herpes simplex and herpes zoster keratouveitis: diagnosis and management. Bull N Y Acad Med 1977;53(8):731–48.
41. Pavan-Langston D, McCulley JP. Herpes zoster dendritic keratitis. Arch Ophthalmol 1973;89(1):25–9.
42. Sanjay S, Huang P, Lavanya R. Herpes zoster ophthalmicus. Curr Treat Options Neurol 2011;13(1):79–91.
43. Seitz B, Heiligenhaus A. "Herpetic keratitis". Various expressions require different therapeutic approaches. Ophthalmologe 2011;108(4):385–95 [quiz: 396–7].
44. Thean JH, Hall AJ, Stawell RJ. Uveitis in Herpes zoster ophthalmicus. Clin Exp Ophthalmol 2001;29(6):406–10.
45. Shaikh S, Ta CN. Evaluation and management of herpes zoster ophthalmicus. Am Fam Physician 2002;66(9):1723–30.
46. Labetoulle M, Colin J. Current concepts in the treatment of herpetic keratitis. J Fr Ophtalmol 2012;35(4):292–307 [in French].
47. Walpita P, Darougar S, Marsh RJ, et al. Development of an immunofluorescence test for the serodiagnosis of herpes zoster ophthalmicus. Br J Ophthalmol 1986; 70(6):431–4.
48. Gurwood AS, Savochka J. Herpes zoster ophthalmicus. Optometry Today 2001;38–41.
49. Sy A, McLeod SD, Cohen EJ, et al. Practice patterns and opinions in the management of recurrent or chronic herpes zoster ophthalmicus. Cornea 2012;31(7): 786–90.
50. Aggarwal S, Cavalcanti BM, Pavan-Langston D. Treatment of pseudodendrites in herpes zoster ophthalmicus with topical ganciclovir 0.15% gel. Cornea 2014; 33(2):109–13.
51. Andrei G, Snoeck R. Herpes simplex virus drug-resistance: new mutations and insights. Curr Opin Infect Dis 2013;26(6):551–60.
52. De Monchy I, Labbe A, Pogorzalek N, et al. Management of herpes zoster neurotrophic ulcer using a new matrix therapy agent (RGTA): a case report. J Fr Ophtalmol 2012;35(3):187.e1–6 [in French].
53. Fashner J, Bell AL. Herpes zoster and postherpetic neuralgia: prevention and management. Am Fam Physician 2011;83(12):1432–7.
54. Gain P, Thuret G, Chiquet C, et al. Facial anesthetic blocks in the treatment of acute pain during ophthalmic zoster. J Fr Ophtalmol 2003;26(1):7–14 [in French].
55. Gumus K, Gire A, Pflugfelder SC. The successful use of Boston ocular surface prosthesis in the treatment of persistent corneal epithelial defect after herpes zoster ophthalmicus. Cornea 2010;29(12):1465–8.
56. Hales CM, Harpaz R, Ortega-Sanchez I, et al. Update on recommendations for use of herpes zoster vaccine. MMWR Morb Mortal Wkly Rep 2014;63(33): 729–31.

57. Marsh RJ, Cooper M. Acyclovir and steroids in herpes zoster keratouveitis. Br J Ophthalmol 1984;68(12):904–5.
58. Marsh RJ, Cooper M. Oral acyclovir in acute herpes zoster. Br Med J (Clin Res Ed) 1987;294(6573):704.
59. Marsh RJ, Cooper M. Ocular surgery in ophthalmic zoster. Eye (Lond) 1989;3(Pt 3):313–7.
60. Marsh RJ, Cooper M. Double-masked trial of topical acyclovir and steroids in the treatment of herpes zoster ocular inflammation. Br J Ophthalmol 1991;75(9): 542–6.
61. Meller D, Thomasen H, Steuhl K. Amniotic membrane transplantation in herpetic corneal infections. Klin Monbl Augenheilkd 2010;227(5):393–9 [in German].
62. Neoh C, Harding SP, Saunders D, et al. Comparison of topical and oral acyclovir in early herpes zoster ophthalmicus. Eye (Lond) 1994;8(Pt 6):688–91.
63. Opstelten W, Zaal MJ. Managing ophthalmic herpes zoster in primary care. BMJ 2005;331(7509):147–51.
64. Pavan-Langston D, Dohlman CH. Boston keratoprosthesis treatment of herpes zoster neurotrophic keratopathy. Ophthalmology 2008;115(2 Suppl):S21–3.
65. Harpaz R, Ortega-Sanchez IR, Seward JF. Prevention of herpes zoster: recommendations of the Advisory Committee on Immunization Practices (ACIP). MMWR Recomm Rep 2008;57(Rr-5):1–30 [quiz: CE2–4].
66. Yawn BP, Wollan PC, St Sauver JL, et al. Herpes zoster eye complications: rates and trends. Mayo Clin Proc 2013;88(6):562–70.
67. Yawn BP, Itzler RF, Wollan PC, et al. Health care utilization and cost burden of herpes zoster in a community population. Mayo Clin Proc 2009;84(9):787–94.
68. Kahloun R, Attia S, Jelliti B, et al. Ocular involvement and visual outcome of herpes zoster ophthalmicus: review of 45 patients from Tunisia, North Africa. J Ophthalmic Inflamm Infect 2014;4:25.
69. Komolafe OO, Ogunleye OT, Fasina OO, et al. African traditional medication and keloid formation in herpes zoster ophthalmicus. Niger J Clin Pract 2011;14(4): 479–81.
70. Tsuda H, Tanaka K. Internal carotid artery involvement in herpes zoster ophthalmicus. Intern Med 2012;51(15):2067–8.
71. Wang CC, Shiang JC, Chen JT, et al. Syndrome of inappropriate secretion of antidiuretic hormone associated with localized herpes zoster ophthalmicus. J Gen Intern Med 2011;26(2):216–20.
72. Zaal MJ, Maudgal PC, Rietveld E, et al. Chronic ocular zoster. Curr Eye Res 1991; 10(Suppl):125–30.
73. Johnson RW, Bouhassira D, Kassianos G, et al. The impact of herpes zoster and post-herpetic neuralgia on quality-of-life. BMC Med 2010;8:37.
74. Womack LW, Liesegang TJ. Complications of herpes zoster ophthalmicus. Arch Ophthalmol 1983;101(1):42–5.
75. Browning WD, McCarthy JP. A case series: herpes simplex virus as an occupational hazard. J Esthet Restor Dent 2012;24(1):61–6.
76. Johnson JA, Bloch KC, Dang BN. Varicella reinfection in a seropositive physician following occupational exposure to localized zoster. Clin Infect Dis 2011;52(7): 907–9.

Uveitis

James P. Dunn, MD

KEYWORDS

- Uveitis • Multidisciplinary management • Ocular inflammatory disease • Scleritis
- Corticosteroids • Immunosuppressive therapy • Biologics

KEY POINTS

- Multidisciplinary management in the diagnosis and management of patients with ocular inflammatory disease is often critical.
- The workup of uveitis or scleritis may reveal an underlying systemic disease; recognition of inflammation by the primary care physician can facilitate prompt referral to a uveitis specialist and improve patient outcomes.
- The primary care physician can assist the ophthalmologist in monitoring for potential side effects of corticosteroids and immunosuppressive drugs, including the newer biologic agents.
- The ophthalmologist in turn can assist the primary care physician in recognizing that active uveitis may suggest incomplete control of preexisting conditions, such as sarcoidosis, ankylosing spondylitis, juvenile rheumatoid arthritis, or vasculitis.

OVERVIEW OF UVEITIS

The uveal tract comprises the iris and ciliary body anteriorly and the choroid posteriorly. Although a strict definition of uveitis, therefore, is limited to inflammation of these tissues, in common usage uveitis also includes inflammation of adjacent tissues, including the cornea, sclera, retina, and even the optic nerve. Multiple structures may be involved (eg, sclerokeratitis, retinochoroiditis).

The Standardization of Uveitis Nomenclature (SUN) Working Group[1] defined types of uveitis by anatomic location and is the most commonly recognized descriptive format used in the uveitis literature. **Table 1** lists the types of uveitis anatomically by the primary site of inflammation location (eg, anterior, intermediate, posterior, and panuveitis). The SUN system also emphasizes the importance of onset (sudden vs insidious), duration (limited vs persistent), and course (acute, recurrent, or chronic) of uveitis (**Table 2**) and provides a grading scale for anterior uveitis. Grading scales for intermediate uveitis based on the amount of vitreous inflammation have also been described. Because these scales require the use of the slit-lamp and indirect ophthalmoscopes, only an ophthalmologist can categorize the uveitis by severity.

Disclosure: The author has no financial disclosures to report.
Uveitis Unit, Retina Division, Wills Eye Hospital, Sidney Kimmel Medical College, Thomas Jefferson University, 840 Walnut Street, Suite 1020, Philadelphia, PA 19107, USA
E-mail address: jpdunn@willseye.org

Prim Care Clin Office Pract 42 (2015) 305–323
http://dx.doi.org/10.1016/j.pop.2015.05.003   **primarycare.theclinics.com**
0095-4543/15/$ – see front matter © 2015 Elsevier Inc. All rights reserved.

Table 1
The SUN anatomic classification of uveitis

Type of Uveitis	Primary Site of Inflammation	Common Manifestations
Anterior	Anterior chamber	Iritis Iridocyclitis
Intermediate	Vitreous	Vitreitis
Posterior	Retina Choroid Optic nerve	Retinitis Choroiditis Retinochoroiditis Chorioretinitis Neuroretinitis
Panuveitis	Anterior chamber, vitreous, retina, choroid, and/or optic nerve	All of the above

Adapted from Jabs DA, Nussenblatt RB, Rosenbaum JT, Standardization of Uveitis Nomenclature Working Group. Standardization of uveitis nomenclature for reporting clinical data: results of the first international workshop. Am J Ophthalmol 2005;140:510; with permission.

Scleritis is categorized as either anterior (eg, diffuse, nodular, or necrotizing) or posterior. Episcleritis is a milder and more superficial form of inflammation.

Other descriptive categorizations are also useful in some cases:

- Infectious versus noninfectious
- Granulomatous versus nongranulomatous
- Unilateral versus bilateral
- Solitary retinal/choroidal lesions versus multifocal
- Purely ocular versus systemic disease association
- Traumatic: blunt force, postoperative, or penetrating
- Uveitis versus pseudouveitis (masquerade syndromes, such as lymphoma)

Symptoms of uveitis vary based on the anatomic location, type of uveitis, duration of disease activity, extent of therapy, and presence or absence of prior sequelae. Common symptoms include blurred or distorted vision, pain, photophobia (light sensitivity), floaters, photopsia (flashing lights), blind spots, and haloes.

Cataract, macular edema, epiretinal membrane (wrinkling of the macula), and glaucoma are the most common complications of uveitis causing visual loss. Other signs

Table 2
The SUN working group descriptors of uveitis

Category	Descriptor	Definition
Onset	Sudden	Rapid onset of symptoms
	Insidious	Gradual onset of symptoms
Duration	Limited	≤3-mo Duration
	Persistent	>3-mo Duration
Course	Acute	Single episode with sudden onset and limited duration
	Recurrent	Repeated episodes separated by inactive periods without treatment ≥3 mo in duration
	Chronic	Persistent uveitis with relapse within 3 mo after discontinuing treatment

Adapted from Jabs DA, Nussenblatt RB, Rosenbaum JT, Standardization of Uveitis Nomen-clature Working Group. Standardization of uveitis nomenclature for reporting clinical data: results of the first international workshop. Am J Ophthalmol 2005;140:511; with permission.

of uveitis include ciliary flush (a violaceous ring around the cornea indicates intraocular inflammation [**Fig. 1**]), corneal/scleral thinning, keratic precipitates (inflammatory deposits on the posterior cornea) (**Fig. 2**), corneal edema, band keratopathy (calcium deposits beneath the corneal epithelium), anterior/posterior synechiae (adhesions of the iris to the cornea or lens, respectively) (**Fig. 3**), hypopyon (a layering of inflammatory cells in the inferior angle), vitreous haze, snowballs (large collections of inflammatory cells in the vitreous), snowbanking (inflammatory exudates over the pars plana), cystoid macular edema (CME), retinal vasculitis, retinal ischemia and/or hemorrhage, retinal/choroidal neovascularization, retinal detachment (exudative or rhegmatogenous), hypotony (low intraocular pressure), and phthisis (a shrunken globe with loss of architectural detail).

Some chronic forms of uveitis are largely asymptomatic, and patients will present only after they develop significant vision. Regular screening is indicated in certain high-risk diseases, such as juvenile rheumatoid arthritis (JRA).[2]

A careful review of systems and external examination is often enough to suggest the correct diagnosis for the primary care physician. Classic examples include

- Chronic anterior uveitis in a 5-year-old girl with a history of JRA presenting with bilateral blurred vision and floaters, irregular pupils, with white or quiet external eyes
- Acute, recurrent HLA-B27–associated anterior uveitis in a 25-year-old patient with ankylosing spondylitis presenting with sudden onset of pain, redness, and light sensitivity photophobia with ciliary flush in one eye
- Panuveitis in a 45-year-old patient with a history of pulmonary sarcoidosis presenting with bilateral blurred vision and floaters
- Intermediate uveitis in a 35-year-old patient with high-risk sexual behavior presenting with bilateral floaters, eye pain, and redness as well as a palmar rash consistent with secondary syphilis
- Anterior scleritis in a 65-year-old patient with recent herpes zoster ophthalmicus presenting with unilateral redness and deep, boring ocular pain

Such concise descriptions can be extremely useful in facilitating referral and treatment in affected patients, particularly in cases in which an underlying systemic disease is suspected or a need for systemic therapy (and, therefore, the potential for adverse drug effects) is likely. Overall, 30% to 45% of uveitis is associated with a systemic disease.[3]

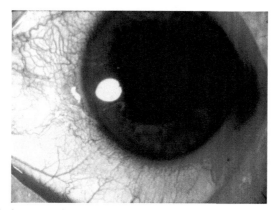

Fig. 1. Ciliary flush. Note the circumlimbal hyperemia that becomes less prominent peripherally.

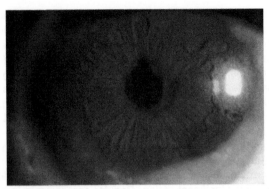

Fig. 2. Sarcoid uveitis with posterior synechiae and peripheral mutton-fat keratic precipitates with corneal haze.

EPIDEMIOLOGY

The incidence and prevalence of uveitis varies based on methodological, age, socioeconomic, racial, sex, genetic, lifestyle, and geographic factors. For example, ocular Behçet disease is much more common in Saudi Arabia than in the United States,[4] and sarcoid-associated uveitis is 3 to 4 times more common in US blacks than whites and is much more common in northern than southern Europe.[5] Various estimates of incidence and prevalence, respectively, in recent US studies range from 25 per 100,000 person-years and 58 per 100,000 persons[6] to 52 per 100,000 person-years and 115 per 100,000 persons, respectively.[7] Among idiopathic (undifferentiated) cases, it is likely that currently unidentified infections (particularly viral)[8] or underreporting of known causes, such as drug-induced uveitis,[9] account for a significant percentage. Toxins may also play a role; Ostheimer and colleagues[10] recently identified a subset of patients in whom tattoo ink seemed to cause uveitis with concurrent induration of the pigmented but not adjacent skin. A history of smoking is significantly associated with all anatomic subtypes of both uveitis and infectious uveitis.[11]

Anterior uveitis comprises more than 90% of cases seen by comprehensive ophthalmologists versus roughly 50% to 60% of anterior uveitis and 10% to 20% each of intermediate uveitis, posterior uveitis, and panuveitis in tertiary uveitis clinics.[12] In

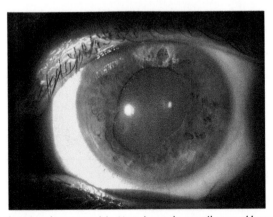

Fig. 3. Herpes simplex virus keratouveitis. Note irregular pupil caused by posterior synechiae and superior iris atrophy.

one study, the mean age at onset of uveitis was 37.2 years with a slight female pre-dominance. Chronic (58.3%), nongranulomatous (77.7%), and noninfectious (83.1%) forms of uveitis were observed most frequently; no identifiable cause was found in 35% of cases.[13]

The incidence of uveitis is lower than in children (roughly 5 per 100,000 person-years), although it does increase with age.[14] Anterior uveitis accounts for more than half of all uveitis seen in a pediatric uveitis tertiary care setting, with intermediate uve-itis more common and posterior uveitis somewhat less common than in adults. Roughly 70% to 80% of pediatric cases are undifferentiated, with JRA the most commonly associated systemic disease.

Scleritis and episcleritis both occur more commonly in women and with increasing age. In one study, the incidence and prevalence of episcleritis was 41 per 100,000 person-years and 53 per 100,000 persons; for scleritis, the incidence was 3 per 100,000 person-years and 5 per 100,000 persons, respectively.[15] About 25% to 35% of patients with episcleritis or scleritis have an associated systemic disease.[16]

ECONOMIC IMPACT OF UVEITIS AND VISUAL LOSS

Uveitis is the fourth leading cause of preventable blindness in the middle-aged popu-lation of the developed world[17,18] and accounts for about 10% to 15% of all blindness, including about 30,000 new cases of blindness yearly in the United States.[19] In addi-tion, the morbidity associated with uveitis causes a disproportionate impact on work-ing adults, as 70% to 90% of patients with uveitis present between 20 to 60 years of age.[18] More than $240 million is spent annually on health care in the United States for patients with uveitis and its consequent morbidity.[17]

PATHOPHYSIOLOGY

Most noninfectious uveitis is thought to be T-cell mediated, predominantly CD4-positive T cells via a Th1 phenotype that results in increased production of interleukin-2, interferon-gamma, and tumor necrosis factor (TNF)–alpha.[20] Nonethe-less, our understanding of the pathophysiology of ocular inflammation is limited; there-fore, most cases are truly undifferentiated.[21] For the clinician, however, it helps to consider the following possible mechanisms:

- Inflammatory
- Infectious
- Traumatic
- Genetic
- Neoplastic
- Ischemic
- Drug induced

There is obviously a substantial overlap between these mechanisms, so that no sin-gle cause of uveitis is likely in noninfectious uveitis. Nonetheless, considering the possible causes of the uveitis and scleritis will help guide the subsequent workup for an underlying systemic disease.

MONITORING FOR COMPLICATIONS

Because one of the most critical factors in the outcome of patients with uveitis is the time from onset of symptoms to referral to a uveitis specialist,[22] a high index of sus-picion is essential in patients with any visual complaints and findings suggestive of uveitis. Furthermore, patients with a history of JRA or Behçet disease, bilateral uveitis, prior cataract surgery, or vision of 20/200 or less at presentation are more likely to develop chronic uveitis warranting more aggressive management than those patients lacking such features[23]; multidisciplinary care is often required in such situations.

Anterior uveitis, intermediate uveitis, posterior uveitis, and panuveitis can all cause numerous ocular complications, with the most common causes of visual loss including cataract, glaucoma, epiretinal membrane, retinal scars, and CME. Furthermore, treatment with corticosteroids increases the risks of cataract, glaucoma, and (with eye drops) infectious keratitis (**Fig. 4**).

Every effort should be made to minimize the risk of cataract and glaucoma because outcomes of surgery for each of these morbidities are less favorable than in patients without uveitis.[24,25]

WORKUP FOR THE PRIMARY CARE PHYSICIAN

The history and physical examination are the most important diagnostic tools for the clinician and will often narrow the differential diagnosis significantly even in the absence of a slit-lamp examination. Some types of uveitis have established diagnostic criteria that help guide the workup, such as JRA-associated uveitis[26] or ocular sarcoidosis.[27] Others have characteristic fundoscopic appearances and angiographic findings (including many of the so-called white dot syndromes[28]) that obviate laboratory testing (**Fig. 5**). A discussion of the approximately 30 diseases associated with uveitis is beyond the scope of this article, but **Table 3** lists some of the more common entities.

Conversely, the ophthalmologist may suspect a systemic disease that the primary care physician can then confirm. In one study of HLA-B27–associated uveitis,[29] 58% of patients had an associated systemic disease, of which more than half had not previously been diagnosed.

The goal is to be parsimonious rather than using a shotgun technique, with an emphasis on distinguishing infectious versus noninfectious disease, recognizing acute versus chronic disease, and avoiding tests with limited positive or negative predictive value, even if their sensitivity and specificity are good.[3,21] For example, if an antinuclear antibody or a purified protein derivative tuberculin skin test is routinely obtained in all patients with uveitis but a low likelihood of systemic lupus erythematosus or tuberculosis (TB), there will be far more false positives than true positives[30]; patients

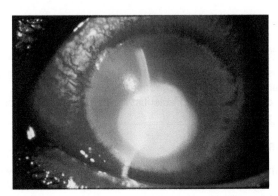

Fig. 4. Candida keratitis secondary to prolonged topical corticosteroid therapy.

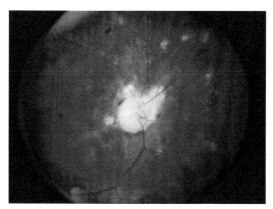

Fig. 5. Advanced birdshot retinopathy. Note the pale optic disk, narrowed retinal arterioles, and scattered chorioretinal scars characteristic of this white dot disorder.

may be subjected to inappropriate and potentially harmful treatment. In some cases, combinations of laboratory tests increase the diagnostic yield, such as urinary β2-microglobulin and serum creatinine in patients with tubulointerstitial nephritis and uveitis.[31]

It is reasonable to obtain a chest radiograph and both fluorescent treponemal antibody absorption test and VDRL in adults with uveitis because sarcoidosis and syphilis can cause virtually any form of uveitis. In other cases, diagnostic studies are

Table 3
Common uveitic diseases

Anatomic Location	Infectious	Noninfectious, Systemic	Noninfectious, Ocular Only
Anterior	• CMV uveitis • HSV uveitis • VZV uveitis • Syphilis • TB • Lyme disease	• juvenile idiopathic arthritis-associated uveitis • Sarcoidosis • HLA-B27–associated uveitis • Multiple sclerosis • TINU • Behçet disease • Multiple sclerosis	• Fuchs' uveitis syndrome • Posttraumatic uveitis
Intermediate	• Syphilis • Lyme disease	• Sarcoidosis • Multiple sclerosis	• Pars planitis
Posterior	• Toxoplasmosis • CMV retinitis • TB • Cat-scratch disease	• Sarcoidosis • CVD-associated vasculitis	• White dot syndromes
Panuveitis	• Syphilis • Acute retinal necrosis • TB	• Sarcoidosis • Behçet disease • V-K-H disease	• Sympathetic ophthalmia

Abbreviations: CMV, cytomegalovirus; CVD, collagen vascular disease; HSV, herpes simplex virus; TB, tuberculosis; TINU, tubulointerstitial nephritis and uveitis; V-K-H, Vogt-Koyanagi-Harada; VZV, varicella zoster virus.
Adapted from Jabs DA, Businiye J. Approach to the diagnosis of the uveitides. Am J Ophthalmol 2013;156:229; with permission.

performed according to the differential diagnosis established with the history and physical examination. Often, the primary care physician will coordinate these tests, which may include

- Serologic evaluation
  - HLA testing (HLA-B27 for seronegative spondyloarthropathies, HLA-A29 for birdshot retinochoroidopathy)
  - Infectious serologies (eg, toxoplasmosis)
  - Autoantibodies (vasculitis)
  - Urinalysis (red blood cells and casts in granulomatosis with polyangiitis [GPA], β2-microglobulinuria in tubulointerstitial nephritis with uveitis)
  - Interferon-gamma releasing assays (eg, QuantiFERON TB Gold [Qiagen, Germantown, MD] testing)
- Radiology and other imaging studies
  - Chest radiograph (sarcoidosis, GPA, TB)
  - Sacroiliac radiographs (seronegative spondyloarthropathies)
  - Computed tomography (CT) abdomen/pelvis (inflammatory bowel disease, Whipple disease)
  - CT chest (sarcoid, TB, GPA)
  - MRI (multiple sclerosis, scleritis)
  - Gallium scan (sarcoidosis)

Ultimately, the goals of the uveitis workup include[21]

- Diagnose a specific disease if possible because of therapeutic and prognostic implications. (For example, some uveitides are self-limited and require no treatment; others are known to be unresponsive to corticosteroids alone and require early intervention with immunosuppressive agents.)
- Diagnose a systemic disease not identified before onset of the uveitis (eg, ankylosing spondylitis[29]).
- Recognize the limitations of laboratory tests.
- Test for those conditions that can present as virtually any form of uveitis (eg, sarcoidosis and syphilis).

TREATMENT

There is no standard regimen for the treatment of any type of uveitis. Therapy is based on the likelihood of efficacy, laterality, anatomic location, previous response and tolerance to therapy, concurrent ocular or systemic disease, patient preference, physician experience, and cost and availability of drugs. A stepwise approach is favored, usually beginning with corticosteroids and progressing to immunosuppressive agents as needed. Most immunosuppressive drugs require 1 to 2 months to achieve full efficacy, so that corticosteroids are necessary early in treatment.[32] Having a specific diagnosis is helpful because it may determine the need for chronic therapy (which often favors corticosteroid-sparing agents) or indicate a disease for which corticosteroids are inadequate therapy. For example, treatment with anti–TNF agents may be considered a first-line option in patients with Behçet disease.[33] Finally, it is important to recognize that Food and Drug Administration (FDA) approval for the treatment of uveitis exists only for corticosteroid eye drops (anterior uveitis) and sustained-release corticosteroid implants (intermediate uveitis, posterior uveitis, and panuveitis); all other forms of corticosteroids and all immunosuppressive agents are used off label.

Randomized controlled clinical uveitis treatment trials have been infrequently published. The relative rarity of uveitis, variations in preferred practice patterns based on training, prior authorization requirements, physician experience, and the fact that different types of uveitis may respond differently to different therapies make it difficult to perform definitive treatment trials.

The goals of therapy, as outlined by expert recommendations,[32,33] include

- Preservation of visual acuity
- Prompt identification of all sources of inflammation
- Zero tolerance toward any degree of inflammation
- Appropriate screening for ocular complications of corticosteroids
- Transition of corticosteroid to immunomodulatory or biologic therapy when corticosteroids are ineffective, not tolerated, or require suppressive dosages of prednisone 10 mg or more daily
- Proper management of both ocular and systemic complications
- Coordination of therapy when systemic disease is associated with uveitis
- Reassessment of diagnostic and treatment options when therapy is ineffective

Corticosteroids can be used as local (topical, periocular, or intravitreal) or systemic (oral or intravenous) forms. Topical corticosteroids are used in the treatment of anterior uveitis and occasionally may be helpful in mild intermediate uveitis. Although there is no standard regimen, most clinicians prefer a use-enough-soon-enough approach, in which the drops are given every 1 to 2 hours during the day, often with a loading dose of one drop every minute for 3 to 5 minutes at bedtime and on awakening. The drops are tapered according to the degree of inflammation, with the long-term goal of discontinuing them altogether. If inflammation persists as the drops are tapered, consideration should be given to initiating corticosteroid-sparing immunosuppressive therapy so as to minimize the risks of glaucoma[34] and cataract.[35] However, the ocular risks in a patient whose uveitis is controlled with chronic, low-dose topical corticosteroids must be balanced against the risks of corticosteroid-sparing drugs.

The efficacy of topical corticosteroids is a function of both transcorneal absorption and potency, with as much as a 20-fold difference in intraocular concentration between different drugs.[36] There is also variable potency of generic forms of corticosteroid suspensions, such as prednisolone acetate, caused by differing sizes of the corticosteroid crystals.[37]

In general, the more potent topical corticosteroids have a greater risk of causing steroid-induced glaucoma, especially in children. Difluprednate 0.05% 4 times daily is comparably effective with prednisolone acetate 1% 8 times daily,[38] which may improve adherence; difluprednate is also an emulsion rather than a suspension, so it does not require shaking. However, it is substantially more expensive than prednisolone acetate. Less potent corticosteroid drops (eg, loteprednol etabonate, dexamethasone, fluorometholone) may not be effective in achieving early control of anterior uveitis but may have a role in patients who need chronic, low-dose therapy to minimize side effects. Combination antibiotic-corticosteroid preparations should not be used in the treatment of noninfectious uveitis to avoid the potential toxicity of the antibiotics (especially aminoglycosides) and because antibiotic prophylaxis is not indicated in the absence of corneal epithelial defects.

Periocular corticosteroids, such as triamcinolone acetonide, can be used as a supplement to topical corticosteroids for severe anterior uveitis but are more commonly used as local therapy for intermediate uveitis and macular edema. As with topical corticosteroids, glaucoma and cataract are common.[39]

Intravitreal corticosteroids can be given in the form of injectable triamcinolone acetonide or sustained-release implants. Only preservative-free triamcinolone injections should be used because of the risk of noninfectious endophthalmitis. The FDA has approved 2 sustained-release corticosteroid implants for treatment of noninfectious intermediate uveitis, posterior uveitis, and panuveitis:

- Retisert is a 0.59 mg fluocinolone acetonide intravitreal implant lasting approximately 30 months; the supporting strut is sutured externally to the sclera with the drug pellet in the vitreous cavity.
- Ozurdex is a free-floating cylinder containing 0.7 mg dexamethasone with a 3- to 6-month duration, implanted by sutureless intravitreal injection.

Both implants avoid the risks of systemic corticosteroids and can reduce the need for immunosuppressive therapy. The fluocinolone implant has a much longer duration of therapy; disadvantages include the need for surgery, glaucoma in up to 60% of patients (roughly half of whom require glaucoma surgery), cataract in greater than 90% of patients within 2 years of implantation, and infection related to exposed sutures or wound leak. The dexamethasone implant can be placed in an office setting, but the procedure must be repeated much more often than the fluocinolone implant. In a small, nonrandomized comparison of the two implants,[40] the dexamethasone implant was comparable with the fluocinolone acetonide implant in preventing recurrence of noninfectious uveitis and in improving inflammation and visual acuity. Rates of cataract progression and need for glaucoma medications, laser, and surgery were higher with the fluocinolone acetonide implant; but the variable time to follow-up between the two groups made comparisons less valid.

The use of steroid-sparing agents is indicated if chronic steroid usage (7.5–10.0 mg or more of prednisone or equivalent daily) is required to control the inflammation; 28% to 59% of patients with noninfectious uveitis will develop visual loss that requires a therapy beyond corticosteroids.[17] For reasons of cost and clinical experience, immunomodulatory therapy (IMT) is usually initiated with traditional immunosuppressive drugs from the following categories:

- Antimetabolites (methotrexate, mycophenolate mofetil or mycophenolate sodium, azathioprine)
- Calcineurin inhibitors (cyclosporine A, tacrolimus)
- Alkylating agents (cyclophosphamide, chlorambucil)

Uveitis is usually controlled in 50% to 70% of cases with these drugs and is generally well tolerated.[32,41] Nonetheless, careful monitoring for side effects (**Table 4**) is necessary. In a randomized trial of systemic antiinflammatory therapy to the fluocinolone implant for intermediate/posterior/panuveitis,[41] mean visual acuity over 24 months improved comparably in the two groups. Systemic therapy with aggressive use of corticosteroid-sparing immunosuppression was well tolerated. Therefore, the choice of therapy should be based on factors other than visual outcomes alone.

A comparison of antimetabolite therapy for uveitis and scleritis suggested that the time to control of ocular inflammation is faster with mycophenolate than with methotrexate; azathioprine therapy had a higher rate of treatment-related side effects compared with the other two agents.[42]

Calcineurin inhibitors are used less frequently than antimetabolites for ocular inflammatory disease. A small randomized controlled study suggested that cyclosporine and tacrolimus are comparably effective, but tacrolimus had a more favorable side effect profile.[43]

The cytotoxic agents are most likely to induce long-term, drug-free remission of uveitis and scleritis but have the least favorable side effect profile of the IMT agents and are used less frequently now that biologic therapy is available.[32,33]

Uveitis   **315**

Table 4
Immunosuppressive drugs and their side effects

Category	Drugs	Common Side Effects
Antimetabolites	Azathioprine Methotrexate Mycophenolate mofetil	Hepatotoxicity, GI upset, fatigue, bone marrow suppression
Calcineurin inhibitors	Cyclosporine-A	Hypertension, chronic kidney disease, tremor, hirsutism, gingivitis, neurologic symptoms
	Tacrolimus	Hypertension, chronic kidney disease, tremor, diabetes, neurologic symptoms, hyperkalemia, hypomagnesemia
Alkylating agents	Chlorambucil	Hemorrhagic cystitis, increased risk malignancies (but not bladder cancer), pancytopenia, sepsis, GI upset
	Cyclophosphamide	Hemorrhagic cystitis; bladder; increased risk malignancies, including bladder cancer; pancytopenia; sepsis; GI upset; alopecia
TNF-alpha inhibitors	Adalimumab Infliximab (Note: etanercept is not recommended for treatment of uveitis)	Increased risk of infection (especially TB), autoimmune disease, demyelinating disease, congestive heart failure, possible increased risk of lymphoma and skin cancer, infusion reactions with infliximab
CD20 inhibitor	Rituximab	Flulike symptoms, nausea, hypotension, anemia, leukopenia, sepsis

Adapted from Jabs DA, Rosenbaum JT, Foster CS, et al. Guidelines for the use of immunosuppressive drugs in patients with ocular inflammatory disorders: recommendations of an expert panel. Am J Ophthalmol 2000;130:492–513; and Levy-Clarke G, Jabs DA, Read RW, et al. Expert panel recommendations for the use of anti-tumor necrosis factor biologic agents in patients with ocular inflammatory disorders. Ophthalmology 2014;121:785–96.

Biologic agents are increasingly used for the treatment of uveitis and its complications when corticosteroids and/or other immunosuppressive drugs are not tolerated or ineffective.[33] These include

- TNF antagonists (adalimumab, infliximab, certolizumab, golimumab, etanercept)
- Anti-CD20 drugs (rituximab)
- Interleukin-6 receptor antagonist (tocilizumab)
- Interleukin-1 receptor antagonist (anakinra)
- Interferon-alpha
- Anti-CD80/86 drugs (blocks costimulatory signals from antigen-presenting cells) (abatacept)
- Vascular endothelial growth factor antagonists (bevacizumab, ranibizumab) (for macular edema)

Among these biologic agents, experience is greatest with the TNF antagonists adalimumab and infliximab. Paradoxically, etanercept may increase the risk of uveitis and scleritis,[44] so that other TNF antagonists are preferred for ocular inflammation.

In cases in which IMT is ineffective, changing from one IMT agent to another, or using combination therapy, may be effective.[45]

Alkylating agents increase the risk of hematologic malignancies, such as leukemia and lymphoma; cyclophosphamide (but not chlorambucil) is associated with hemorrhagic cystitis and an increased risk of bladder cancer. Antimetabolites, daclizumab,

TNF antagonists, and calcineurin inhibitors do not seem to increase cancer risk to a degree that outweighs the expected benefits of therapy. Monitoring for skin cancer is recommended for highly sun-exposed patients.[46]

Oral nonsteroidal antiinflammatory drugs (NSAIDS) are first-line agents in the treatment of many types of noninfectious scleritis[47] but have a minimal role in the treatment of uveitis. The different NSAIDS vary in their potency; ibuprofen is usually insufficient therapeutically except at high doses that increase the risk of gastrointestinal side effects. Many clinicians prefer flurbiprofen, ketoprofen, diclofenac, or indomethacin instead. Side effects include gastrointestinal upset, gastric ulceration, and renal insufficiency. Subconjunctival or oral corticosteroids and immunosuppressive drugs can be used if NSAIDS are ineffective or not tolerated.

OUTCOMES

The outcomes seem to be improving in patients with uveitis over time. A large study from 2014 found that average acuity remained stable for patients with both anterior uveitis (20/30 at baseline to 20/33 at 10 years) and nonanterior uveitis (20/50 at baseline to 20/47 at 10 years).[48] The investigators postulated that the use of aggressive topical, periocular, and oral corticosteroid therapy; traditional immunosuppressive drugs, such as mycophenolate mofetil; and biologic agents accounted for the favorable outcomes. Nonetheless, 19% of patients had some vision loss, emphasizing the importance of careful follow-up; patients required ophthalmic examination an average of 6 times per year, and one-third required surgery for uveitis-related complications.

In general, anterior uveitis has the best visual prognosis and posterior/panuveitis the worst; but many factors contribute to outcome. For example, macular scarring and macular edema are much more common in intermediate uveitis, posterior uveitis, and panuveitis.[48] Other poor prognostic features include development of glaucoma,[22] presence of macular edema,[49] epiretinal membrane,[50] and failure to initiate immunosuppressive therapy.[51] One of the most important and underappreciated risk factors for visual loss is delay in presentation to a uveitis subspecialist.[22] Demographic features can be associated with adverse outcomes. (For example, children and blacks are at increased risk of corticosteroid-induced glaucoma.[34]) However, it is important to identify potentially treatable risk factors, such as smoking.[11]

INFECTIOUS UVEITIS

An extended discussion of infectious uveitis is beyond the scope of this article. The most common causes include toxoplasmosis,[52] viral retinitis (cytomegalovirus, herpes simplex virus, and varicella zoster virus),[53,54] syphilis,[55] TB,[56] Lyme borreliosis,[57] and cat-scratch disease.[58] Uveitis in human immunodeficiency virus (HIV)–infected patients with no other identifiable cause has been reported rarely, but HIV testing as part of the workup of nonspecific uveitis is not recommended.[59]

Diagnosis of these various entities is often made on clinical grounds, with laboratory tests used to support the clinician's suspicion. For example, classic toxoplasmosis retinochoroiditis is supported by a positive toxoplasma immunoglobulin G (IgG) (or in acute disease, IgM); but because the prevalence of a positive IgG titer in asymptomatic adults is high, the test carries a low specificity. On the other hand, a negative IgM and IgG titer virtually rules out the possibility of toxoplasmosis, so that serologic testing has a much higher predictive negative value than predictive positive value.[52] Similarly, the diagnosis of ocular Lyme borreliosis cannot be made by a positive Lyme IgG alone; concurrent extraocular findings, endemic exposure, and a confirmatory Western blot test are also critical diagnostically.[57]

Viral retinitis may be diagnosed by polymerase chain reaction (PCR) testing from ocular fluids.[54] Necrotizing herpetic retinopathy (acute retinal necrosis or progressive outer retinal necrosis) is usually caused by varicella zoster or herpes simplex virus in immunocompetent individuals; cytomegalovirus (CMV) is the most common cause in immunocompromised patients, especially those with advanced HIV/AIDS. Although these infections can be treated with intravitreal (off-label) antivirals, such as foscarnet or ganciclovir, it is especially critical to treat both the underlying immunosuppression and CMV infection with highly active antiretroviral therapy and systemic anti-CMV therapy because ocular involvement indicates systemic CMV viremia; mortality is increased if only local anti-CMV therapy is used.[60] Anti-CMV therapy can usually be discontinued if there is a sustained increase in the CD4+ T-cell count to greater than 100/mL. Patients with CMV retinitis and a good response to highly active antiretroviral therapy may develop a syndrome called immune recovery uveitis that includes uveitis, macular edema, and/or epiretinal membrane after the retinitis is inactive.[61] Treatment includes oral or periocular corticosteroids; increasing or resuming anti-CMV therapy is not effective.

CMV can also cause a chronic anterior uveitis without retinitis in immunocompetent individuals and should be considered in patients who fail to respond to topical corticosteroids; PCR testing of anterior chamber fluid is diagnostic.[62] It is likely that PCR testing from ocular fluids will become helpful in the diagnosis of a variety of emerging infections causing uveitis, such as chikungunya and West Nile virus.[8]

PREGNANCY AND UVEITIS

Although individual cases vary, in general pregnancy tends to ameliorate uveitis, particularly in the third trimester.[63] However, disease activity often increases post partum, so that treatment may again require adjustment. Corticosteroid implants are a useful option for women with uveitis who are pregnant or considering becoming pregnant, thereby minimizing risk to the fetus.[64] Contrary to popular belief, pregnancy is not associated with an increased risk of recurrence of ocular toxoplasmosis.[65]

THE ROLE OF THE PRIMARY CARE PHYSICIAN

Effective collaboration between the primary care physician and the ophthalmologist is critical in the diagnosis and management of patients with uveitis. The goals of collaborate care should be to

- Identify systemic diseases, including infections
- Identify and minimize side effects of therapy, both ocular and systemic
- Ensure timely follow-up with care providers
- Consider the possibility of drug-induced uveitis

Systemic corticosteroids and immunosuppressive drugs require regular monitoring, based on evidence-based recommendations from a multidisciplinary panel of ophthalmologists, pediatricians, and rheumatologists with expertise in ocular inflammatory disease.[32]

CORTICOSTEROIDS

Corticosteroids (prednisone, prednisolone) can cause hyperglycemia/diabetes mellitus, hypertension, myopathy, pancreatitis, Cushingoid changes, mood swings (including depression and psychosis), agitation, osteoporosis, lipid abnormalities, atherosclerosis, delayed wound healing, easy bruising, and infection. Children treated with corticosteroids may have delayed pubertal growth.[32] Gastric ulceration is uncommon unless concurrent NSAIDs are used, so that routine use of H2 blockers or proton pump inhibitors is not usually necessary.[32] High-dose oral corticosteroids (eg, prednisone 60–80 mg daily) should be used for no more 1 month and dosages of greater than 20 mg daily for more than 6 months because of a 15% to 20% risk of ischemic necrosis of bone (INB).[66] Chronic doses of prednisone at a dose of less than 10 mg/d are generally tolerated well, but the goal should always be the minimum amount necessary to control the uveitis.

Conversely, topical ophthalmic medications may have systemic side effects; the drops dissolve in the tear film, which drains through the nasolacrimal system and allows absorption across the nasal mucosa. Prolonged use of corticosteroid eye drops can cause growth suppression in children.[67] Primary care physicians should strive to list all ophthalmic drops in a patient's medication profile.

Unfortunately, a recent survey of uveitis specialists found that 75% of respondents were either not aware of or did not follow treatment guidelines for the use of oral corticosteroids that recommend the use of corticosteroid-sparing agents if control of uveitis cannot be achieved with 10 mg/d or less of prednisone within 3 months,[68] further emphasizing the important role the primary physician can play in management of these patients. Monitoring should include the following[32]:

- Monitoring of blood pressure and blood glucose every 3 months
- Bone mineral density evaluations and blood cholesterol and lipid testing annually
- Supplemental calcium 1500 mg and vitamin D 800 IU daily
- Replacement of the sex hormones if decreased or if postmenopausal
- Weight-bearing exercises for all who take chronic oral corticosteroids (particularly in the first 6 months of glucocorticoid therapy when the bone loss is the greatest)

Intravenous corticosteroids are sometimes used as initial pulse therapy (eg, methylprednisolone succinate 1 g daily[32] 3 consecutive days, followed by high-dose oral therapy). Intravenous corticosteroids are not associated with INB[66] but should be given over at least 30 minutes to reduce the risk of arrhythmia, cardiovascular collapse, myocardial infarction, and severe infection.[32]

DRUG-INDUCED UVEITIS AND SCLERITIS

Potential causes of drug-induced uveitis and scleritis include bisphosphonates (scleritis, anterior uveitis, conjunctivitis), chemotherapy (uveitis), rifabutin (anterior uveitis), sulfonamides (anterior uveitis), and vaccinations for hepatitis B and varicella zoster virus (anterior uveitis).[9] Etanercept may cause uveitis, scleritis, and retinal vasculitis.[44] First-time use of oral moxifloxacin and ciprofloxacin, but not levofloxacin, increases the risk of uveitis with pigmentary dispersion and atonic pupils.[69] Fewer than 1% of all cases of uveitis are attributed to adverse drug reactions (ADR); but the rarity of the disease, the failure in many cases to fulfill the Naranjo criteria for possible ADR, and the fact that some drug-induced uveitis may be attributed to the disease the drug is supposed to treat for (eg, etanercept for ocular inflammatory disease) may contribute to underreporting.[9]

For most drugs, regular monitoring is not recommended; but prompt referral to an ophthalmologist is warranted if ocular inflammatory disease develops while on therapy. Most of these adverse drug reactions will resolve with temporary cessation of the drug along with topical and/or oral corticosteroid therapy; but in some cases, permanent cessation of the causative drug is necessary to prevent severe worsening of inflammation with rechallenge.

LOW VISION

Patients with visual impairment of any cause have a broad range of physical and mental health problems, including exacerbation of comorbidities, such as orthopedic or psychiatric disease.[70] Depression and suicide are more common in visually impaired patients, yet ophthalmologists frequently fail to recognize depression or to recommend treatment. It is important to take advantage of low-vision rehabilitation services and to ask about symptoms of depression early in the course of a disease in which permanent loss of vision (not simply blindness) is present or likely to occur. Intervention may allow affected patients to resume driving, reduce dependence on others, regain some activities of daily living, and improve quality of life.

FINAL COMMENTS

Multidisciplinary management in the diagnosis and management of patients with ocular inflammatory disease is often critical. The workup of uveitis or scleritis may reveal an underlying systemic disease. Recognition of inflammation by the primary care physician can facilitate prompt referral to a uveitis specialist and improve patient outcomes. The primary care physician can assist the ophthalmologist in monitoring for potential side effects of corticosteroids and immunosuppressive drugs, including the newer biologic agents. The ophthalmologist in turn can assist the primary care physician in recognizing that active uveitis may suggest incomplete control of preexisting conditions, such as sarcoidosis, ankylosing spondylitis, JRA, or vasculitis.

REFERENCES

1. Jabs DA, Nussenblatt RB, Rosenbaum JT, Standardization of Uveitis Nomenclature Working Group. Standardization of uveitis nomenclature for reporting clinical data: results of the first international workshop. Am J Ophthalmol 2005;140: 509–16.
2. Heiligenhaus A, Niewerth M, Ganser G, et al, German Uveitis in Childhood Study Group. Prevalence and complications of uveitis in juvenile idiopathic arthritis in a population-based nation-wide study in Germany: suggested modification of the current screening guidelines. Rheumatology (Oxford) 2007;46:1015–9.
3. Harman LE, Margo CE, Roetzheim RG. Uveitis: the collaborative diagnostic evaluation. Am Fam Physician 2014;90:711–6.
4. Arevalo JF, Lasave AF, Al Jindan MY, et al, KKESH Uveitis Survey Study Group. Uveitis in Behçet disease in a tertiary center over 25 years: the KKESH Uveitis Survey Study Group. Am J Ophthalmol 2015;159:177–84.
5. Bonfioli AA, Orefice F. Sarcoidosis. Semin Ophthalmol 2005;20:177–82.
6. Acharya NR, Tham VM, Esterberg E, et al. Incidence and prevalence of uveitis: results from the Pacific Ocular Inflammation Study. JAMA Ophthalmol 2013; 131:1405–12.
7. Gritz DC, Wong IG. Incidence and prevalence of uveitis in Northern California; the Northern California Epidemiology of Uveitis Study. Ophthalmology 2004;111: 491–500.
8. Khairallah M, Kahloun R. Ocular manifestations of emerging infectious diseases. Curr Opin Ophthalmol 2013;24:574–80.
9. Cordero-Coma M, Salazar-Méndez R, Garzo-García I, et al. Drug-induced uveitis. Expert Opin Drug Saf 2015;14:111–26.
10. Ostheimer TA, Burkholder BM, Leung TG, et al. Tattoo-associated uveitis. Am J Ophthalmol 2014;158:637–43.

11. Lin P, Loh AR, Margolis TP, et al. Cigarette smoking as a risk factor for uveitis. Ophthalmology 2010;117:585–90.
12. McCannel CA, Holland GN, Helm CJ, et al. Causes of uveitis in the general practice of ophthalmology. UCLA Community-Based Uveitis Study Group. Am J Ophthalmol 1996;121:35–46.
13. Rodriguez A, Calonge M, Pedroza-Seres M, et al. Referral patterns of uveitis in a tertiary eye care center. Arch Ophthalmol 1996;114:593–9.
14. Edelsten C, Reddy MA, Stanford MR, et al. Visual loss associated with pediatric uveitis in English primary and referral centers. Am J Ophthalmol 2003;135: 676–80.
15. Honik G, Wong IG, Gritz DC. Incidence and prevalence of episcleritis and scleritis in Northern California. Cornea 2013;32:1562–6.
16. Sainz de la Maza M, Molina N, Gonzalez-Gonzalez LA, et al. Clinical characteristics of a large cohort of patients with scleritis and episcleritis. Ophthalmology 2012;119:43–50.
17. Nguyen QD, Callanan D, Dugel P, et al. Treating chronic noninfectious posterior segment uveitis: the impact of cumulative damage: proceedings of an expert panel roundtable discussion. Retina 2006;26(Suppl 8):1–16.
18. Suttorp-Schulten MS, Rothova A. The possible impact of uveitis in blindness: a literature survey. Br J Ophthalmol 1996;80:844–8.
19. Nussenblatt RB. The natural course of uveitis. Int Ophthalmol 1990;141:303–8.
20. Durrani OM, Meads CA, Murray PI. Uveitis: a potentially blinding disease. Ophthalmologica 2004;218:223–36.
21. Jabs DA, Busingye J. Approach to the diagnosis of the uveitides. Am J Ophthalmol 2013;156:228–36.
22. Dana MR, Merayo-Lloves J, Schaumberg DA, et al. Prognosticators for visual outcome in sarcoid uveitis. Ophthalmology 1996;103:1846–53.
23. Artornsombudh P, Pistilli M, Foster CS, et al. Factors predictive of remission of new-onset anterior uveitis. Ophthalmology 2014;121:778–84.
24. Mehta S, Linton MM, Kempen JH. Outcomes of cataract surgery in patients with uveitis: a systematic review and meta-analysis. Am J Ophthalmol 2014;158:676–92.
25. Shimizu A, Maruyama K, Yokoyama Y, et al. Characteristics of uveitic glaucoma and evaluation of its surgical treatment. Clin Ophthalmol 2014;8:2383–9.
26. Tugal-Tutkun I, Quartier P, Bodaghi B. Disease of the year: juvenile idiopathic arthritis-associated uveitis–classification and diagnostic approach. Ocul Immunol Inflamm 2014;22:56–63.
27. Herbort CP, Rao NA, Mochizuki M, Members of Scientific Committee of First International Workshop on Ocular Sarcoidosis. International criteria for the diagnosis of ocular sarcoidosis: results of the first International Workshop on Ocular Sarcoidosis (IWOS). Ocul Immunol Inflamm 2009;17:160–9.
28. Matsumoto Y, Haen SP, Spaide RF. The white dot syndromes. Compr Ophthalmol Update 2007;8:179–200 [discussion: 203–4].
29. Tay-Kearney ML, Schwam BL, Lowder C, et al. Clinical features and associated systemic diseases of HLA-B27 uveitis. Am J Ophthalmol 1996;121:47–56.
30. Rosenbaum JT, Wernick R. The utility of routine screening of patients with uveitis for systemic lupus erythematosus or tuberculosis. A Bayesian analysis. Arch Ophthalmol 1990;108:1291–3.
31. Hettinga YM, Scheerlinck LM, Lilien MR, et al. The value of measuring urinary β2-microglobulin and serum creatinine for detecting tubulointerstitial nephritis and uveitis syndrome in young patients with uveitis. JAMA Ophthalmol 2015;133: 140–5.

32. Jabs DA, Rosenbaum JT, Foster CS, et al. Guidelines for the use of immunosuppressive drugs in patients with ocular inflammatory disorders: recommendations of an expert panel. Am J Ophthalmol 2000;130:492–513.
33. Levy-Clarke G, Jabs DA, Read RW, et al. Expert panel recommendations for the use of anti-tumor necrosis factor biologic agents in patients with ocular inflammatory disorders. Ophthalmology 2014;121:785–96.
34. Friedman DS, Holbrook JT, Ansari H, et al, MUST Research Group. Risk of elevated intraocular pressure and glaucoma in patients with uveitis: results of the Multicenter Uveitis Steroid Treatment Trial. Ophthalmology 2013;120:1571–9.
35. Thorne JE, Woreta FA, Dunn JP, et al. Risk of cataract development among children with juvenile idiopathic arthritis-related uveitis treated with topical corticosteroids. Ophthalmology 2010;117:1436–41.
36. McGhee CN, Dean S, Danesh-Meyer H. Locally administered ocular corticosteroids: benefits and risks. Drug Saf 2002;25:33–55.
37. Roberts CW, Nelson PL. Comparative analysis of prednisolone acetate suspensions. J Ocul Pharmacol Ther 2007;23:182–7.
38. Sheppard JD, Toyos MM, Kempen JH, et al. Difluprednate 0.05% versus prednisolone acetate 1% for endogenous anterior uveitis: a phase III, multicenter, randomized study. Invest Ophthalmol Vis Sci 2014;55:2993–3002.
39. Sen HN, Vitale S, Gangaputra SS, et al. Periocular corticosteroid injections in uveitis: effects and complications. Ophthalmology 2014;121:2275–86.
40. Arcinue CA, Cerón OM, Foster CS. A comparison between the fluocinolone acetonide (Retisert) and dexamethasone (Ozurdex) intravitreal implants in uveitis. J Ocul Pharmacol Ther 2013;29:501–7.
41. Multicenter Uveitis Steroid Treatment (MUST) Trial Research Group, Kempen JH, Altaweel MM, et al. Randomized comparison of systemic anti-inflammatory therapy versus fluocinolone acetonide implant for intermediate, posterior, and panuveitis: the multicenter uveitis steroid treatment trial. Ophthalmology 2011;118:1916–26.
42. Galor A, Jabs DA, Leder HA, et al. Comparison of antimetabolite drugs as corticosteroid-sparing therapy for noninfectious ocular inflammation. Ophthalmology 2008;115:1826–32.
43. Murphy CC, Greiner K, Plskova J, et al. Cyclosporine vs tacrolimus therapy for posterior and intermediate uveitis. Arch Ophthalmol 2005;123:634–41.
44. Gaujoux-Viala C, Giampietro C, Gaujoux T, et al. Scleritis: a paradoxical effect of etanercept? Etanercept-associated inflammatory eye disease. J Rheumatol 2012;39:233–9.
45. Joshi L, Talat L, Yaganti S, et al. Outcomes of changing immunosuppressive therapy after treatment failure in patients with noninfectious uveitis. Ophthalmology 2014;121:1119–24.
46. Kempen JH, Gangaputra S, Daniel E, et al. Long-term risk of malignancy among patients treated with immunosuppressive agents for ocular inflammation: a critical assessment of the evidence. Am J Ophthalmol 2008;146:802–12.
47. Beardsley RM, Suhler EB, Rosenbaum JT, et al. Pharmacotherapy of scleritis: current paradigms and future directions. Expert Opin Pharmacother 2013;14:411–24.
48. Tomkins-Netzer O, Talat L, Bar A, et al. Long-term clinical outcome and causes of vision loss in patients with uveitis. Ophthalmology 2014;121:2387–92.
49. Levin MH, Pistilli M, Daniel E, et al, Systemic Immunosuppressive Therapy for Eye Diseases Cohort Study. Incidence of visual improvement in uveitis cases with visual impairment caused by macular edema. Ophthalmology 2014;121:588–95.

50. Lehpamer B, Moshier E, Pahk P, et al. Epiretinal membranes in uveitic macular edema: effect on vision and response to therapy. Am J Ophthalmol 2014;157: 1048–55.
51. Gregory AC 2nd, Kempen JH, Daniel EK, et al, Systemic Immunosuppressive Therapy for Eye Diseases Cohort Study Research Group. Risk factors for loss of visual acuity among patients with uveitis associated with juvenile idiopathic arthritis: the Systemic Immunosuppressive Therapy for Eye Diseases Study. Ophthalmology 2013;120:186–92.
52. Kijlstra A, Petersen E. Epidemiology, pathophysiology, and the future of ocular toxoplasmosis. Ocul Immunol Inflamm 2014;22:138–47.
53. Jabs DA, Ahuja A, Van Natta M, et al, Studies of the Ocular Complications of AIDS Research Group. Comparison of treatment regimens for cytomegalovirus retinitis in patients with AIDS in the era of highly active antiretroviral therapy. Ophthalmology 2013;120:1262–70.
54. Wong RW, Jumper JM, McDonald HR, et al. Emerging concepts in the management of acute retinal necrosis. Br J Ophthalmol 2013;97:545–52.
55. Moradi A, Salek S, Daniel E, et al. Clinical features and incidence rates of ocular complications in patients with ocular syphilis. Am J Ophthalmol 2015;159: 334–43.
56. Gupta A, Sharma A, Bansal R, et al. Classification of intraocular tuberculosis. Ocul Immunol Inflamm 2015;23:7–13.
57. Mikkilä HO, Seppälä IJ, Viljanen MK, et al. The expanding clinical spectrum of ocular Lyme borreliosis. Ophthalmology 2000;107:581–7.
58. Kalogeropoulos C, Koumpoulis I, Mentis A, et al. Bartonella and intraocular inflammation: a series of cases and review of literature. Clin Ophthalmol 2011; 5:817–29.
59. Rose-Nussbaumer J, Goldstein DA, Thorne JE, et al. Uveitis in human immunodeficiency virus-infected persons with CD4+ T-lymphocyte count over 200 cells/mL. Clin Experiment Ophthalmol 2014;42:118–25.
60. Jabs DA, Holbrook JT, Van Natta ML, et al, Studies of Ocular Complications of AIDS Research Group. Risk factors for mortality in patients with AIDS in the era of highly active antiretroviral therapy. Ophthalmology 2005;112:771–9.
61. Nguyen QD, Kempen JH, Bolton SG, et al. Immune recovery uveitis in patients with AIDS and cytomegalovirus retinitis after highly active antiretroviral therapy. Am J Ophthalmol 2000;129:634–9.
62. Woo JH, Lim WK, Ho SL, et al. Characteristics of cytomegalovirus uveitis in immunocompetent patients. Ocul Immunol Inflamm 2014. [Epub ahead of print].
63. Chiam NP, Lim LL. Uveitis and gender: the course of uveitis in pregnancy. J Ophthalmol 2014;2014:401915.
64. Ozzello DJ, Palestine AG. Factors affecting therapeutic decisions in intermediate and posterior uveitis. Am J Ophthalmol 2015;159:213–20.
65. Braakenburg AM, Crespi CM, Holland GN, et al. Recurrence rates of ocular toxoplasmosis during pregnancy. Am J Ophthalmol 2014;157:767–73.
66. Felson DT, Anderson JJ. Across-study evaluation of association between steroid dose and bolus steroids and avascular necrosis of bone. Lancet 1987;1(8538): 902–5.
67. Wolthers OD. Growth suppression caused by corticosteroid eye drops. J Pediatr Endocrinol Metab 2011;24:393–4.
68. Nguyen QD, Hatef E, Kayen B, et al. A cross-sectional study of the current treatment patterns in noninfectious uveitis among specialists in the United States. Ophthalmology 2011;118:184–90.

69. Eadie B, Etminan M, Mikelberg FS. Risk for uveitis with oral moxifloxacin: a comparative safety study. JAMA Ophthalmol 2015;133:81–4.
70. Tasman W, Rovner B. Age-related macular degeneration: treating the whole patient. Arch Ophthalmol 2004;122:648–9.

Conjunctivitis

Susana A. Alfonso, MD, MHCM[a],*, Jonie D. Fawley, PA-C, MPAS[a],
Xiaoqin Alexa Lu, MD[b]

KEYWORDS

- Conjunctivitis • Acute conjunctivitis • Chronic conjunctivitis • Viral conjunctivitis
- Bacterial conjunctivitis • Allergic conjunctivitis

KEY POINTS

- Conjunctivitis is the most common cause of red eye in primary care.
- The 3 most common types of conjunctivitis are viral, allergic, and bacterial, and they can present in either acute or chronic forms; the age of the patient, time of year and physical examination findings are paramount to distinguish the different types of conjunctivitis.
- Distinguishing between acute viral and bacterial conjunctivitis remains difficult. Patients with prolonged symptoms, poor response to initial management, or evidence of severe disease should be referred to ophthalmology for consultation.

INTRODUCTION

Conjunctivitis is a common complaint in primary care. It affects all ages and socioeconomic classes. Approximately 70% of patients with acute conjunctivitis present to their primary care provider or an urgent care center rather than to an ophthalmologist.[1] Research data have shown that 1% of all primary care office visits are related to conjunctivitis, which affects 6 million people annually in the United States.[2,3] The economic impact is significant in terms of the cost of medical visits, cost of treatment, and lost work productivity. Bacterial conjunctivitis, which comprises about 50% of all cases of conjunctivitis, costs an estimated $377 million to $875 million annually in the United States.[4]

Acute conjunctivitis is usually a self-limiting condition that rarely causes permanent loss of vision. However, it is important to rule out other sight-threatening red eye diseases. Primary care providers need to be familiar with common differentials for the cause of a red eye (**Box 1**). Appropriate decision making for a timely referral to an ophthalmologist is paramount to ensure quality patient care (**Box 2**).

[a] Department of Family and Preventive Medicine, Emory Family Medicine at Dunwoody, Emory University School of Medicine, 4500 North Shallowford Road, Dunwoody, GA 30338, USA;
[b] Department of Ophthalmology, Emory Eye Clinic, Emory University School of Medicine, 1365 Clifton Road, Building B, Atlanta, GA 30322, USA
* Corresponding author.
E-mail address: salfons@emory.edu

Prim Care Clin Office Pract 42 (2015) 325–345
http://dx.doi.org/10.1016/j.pop.2015.05.001
0095-4543/15/$ – see front matter © 2015 Elsevier Inc. All rights reserved.

Box 1
Common differential diagnosis of red eye

1. Conjunctivitis

2. Episcleritis and scleritis

3. Corneal ulcer, abrasion, or foreign body

4. Iritis

5. Glaucoma

6. Subconjunctival hematoma

7. Chemical/flash burns

8. Dry eye

9. Blepharitis

A practical and systematic approach is needed to accurately diagnose conjunctivitis. This approach includes a medical history, a detailed ocular history, an ocular examination, a physical examination, and laboratory studies.[5] An ocular history includes details about the type of discharge, presence of pain, itching, blurred vision, photophobia, corneal opacity, and eyelid characteristics. An ocular examination includes measured visual acuity, pupillary responses, extraocular motility, confrontation visual fields, an external eye examination, and a slit-lamp examination. An ocular examination in the primary care setting is limited because of lack of a slit lamp. However, useful clinical findings such as presence and type of discharge, conjunctival injection, or hypertrophy may be obtained with a simple penlight.[6]

DEFINITION

The conjunctiva is a transparent lubricating mucous membrane that covers the surface of the globe (bulbar) and the undersurface of the eyelid (palpebral) **(Fig. 1)**. Conjunctivitis is inflammation or infection of the conjunctiva. It may be infectious or noninfectious.

Infectious conjunctivitis can have diverse causes, such as bacterial, viral, chlamydial, fungal, and parasitic. Causes of noninfectious conjunctivitis include allergens, toxicities, and irritants. Common bacterial pathogens include of *Staphylococcus aureus*, *Streptococcus pneumoniae*, *Haemophilus influenzae*, *Neisseria gonorrhoeae*, *Chlamydia trachomatis*, and diphtheria. Common viral agents include adenovirus,

---

Box 2
When to refer to ophthalmology

1. History of a foreign body or trauma

2. Ciliary flush

3. Asymmetric or nonreactive pupil

4. Copious, rapidly progressive discharge

5. Qualitative loss in visual acuity

6. Inability to open eye or keep it open

7. Corneal opacity

8. Marked pain or photophobia

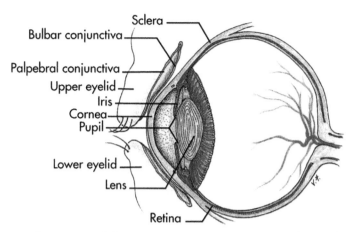

Fig. 1. The anterior segment of the eye. *From* Potter PA, Perry AG. Fundamentals of nursing. 7th edition. St Louis (MO): Mosby; 2009; with permission.

herpes simplex, herpes zoster, and enterovirus. Allergic conjunctivitis encompasses conditions to include seasonal allergic conjunctivitis, perennial allergic conjunctivitis, vernal keratoconjunctivitis (VKC), atopic keratoconjunctivitis (AKC), and giant papillary conjunctivitis. Examples of toxin-induced and irritant-induced conjunctivitis include contact lens–related keratoconjunctivitis, floppy eyelid syndrome, and medication-induced keratoconjunctivitis.

Conjunctivitis can be further divided into acute or chronic types. Acute conjunctivitis is characterized by onset within 3 to 4 weeks of the presentation and chronic is defined as more than 4 weeks in duration.[7]

A distinction between acute and chronic conjunctivitis can be drawn from an assessment of the discharge appearance, physical examination findings, and associated symptoms (**Table 1**).

PREVALENCE AND INCIDENCE

The prevalence of conjunctivitis varies according to the underlying cause, which may be influenced by the patient's age, as well as the season of the year.[6] Allergic conjunctivitis is the most frequent overall cause, affecting 15% to 40% of the population, and

Table 1
Symptom criteria

Symptoms	Allergic Conjunctivitis	Bacterial Conjunctivitis	Viral Conjunctivitis
Appearance of eye discharge	White stringy mucoid	Mucopurulent	Watery
Presence of erythema	Mild to moderate	Moderate to severe	Mild to moderate
Pruritus	Moderate to severe	None to mild	Mild to moderate
Bilateral eye involvement	Common	Unilateral initially	Rare
Presence of lymphadenopathy	None	Rare	Common
Upper respiratory coinfection	None	Rare	Common

Adapted from Cronau H, Kankanala RR, Mauger T. Diagnosis and management of red eye in primary care. Am Fam Physician 2010;81(2):139.

is observed most frequently in the spring and summer.[8] Approximately 20% to 70% of infectious conjunctivitis is thought to be viral and 65% to 90% of viral conjunctivitis is caused by adenovirus and is most prevalent in the summer.[6] Bacterial conjunctivitis is the second most common cause of infectious conjunctivitis and is responsible for most cases in children. It is most frequently observed from December to April.[7] *N gonorrhoeae* is the most common bacterial pathogen in neonates, *H influenzae* is most common in infants and toddlers, and *S aureus* is most common in school-aged children and adults[5] (**Box 3**).

Patient education and hand washing are essential to preventing the spread of contagious conjunctivitis. Conjunctivitis is associated with several conditions and comorbidites (**Box 4**).

Physical Examination

Obtaining the visual acuity of the patient is the first step in assessing the severity of the condition. Visual acuity can be obtained in a primary care setting with the patient wearing current glasses, if applicable, and holding a near vision card 41 cm (16 inches) away from the face. In patients more than 45 years of age, reading glasses might be required for near vision. The pupils should be assessed for equality and reactivity to light. If abnormal, the patient should be referred to ophthalmology emergently (see **Box 2**).

It is important to evaluate the periorbital area for signs of swelling and erythema that might indicate orbital or periorbital cellulitis. The eyelid skin and lashes should be examined for signs of vesicular lesions, discharge or blepharitis, and loss of lashes. Loss of eye lashes could indicate sebaceous gland carcinoma, whereas vesicular lesions can point to herpetic viruses as the cause of inflammation.

The next step of the examination is to recognize the different types of discharge: purulent, mucopurulent, or watery. Purulent discharge is usually hyperacute and reforms as soon as it is cleared from the eye. Mucopurulent discharge is adherent to the eyelashes and has a higher mucus content (**Fig. 4**). Watery discharge is mostly clear and can be copious (**Fig. 5**).

The examiner should be comfortable pulling on the lower lid and everting the upper lid to examine the palpebral conjunctiva. The presence of follicles, papillae, or membranes is another important tool in diagnosis. Follicles are small yellowish elevations of lymphocytes and are usually seen in the lower cul-de-sac at the junction of the palpebral and bulbar conjunctiva (**Fig. 6**). A follicular response is usually seen in conjunctivitis caused by adenovirus and chlamydia. Papillae are small conjunctival elevations with central vessels and can be readily appreciated under the superior tarsal conjunctiva (**Fig. 11**). A papillary reaction could indicate the presence of allergic conjunctivitis and contact lens intolerance. Conjunctival membranes can form in cases of severe infection. The membrane consists of a yellow to whitish colored fibrin layer that is

---

Box 3
Risk factors

1. Age: children have the highest incidence
2. Seasonal allergies
3. Exposure to known allergens
4. Sharing towels or linens with a person who has conjunctivitis
5. Use of contact lenses

Box 4
Comorbidities

1. Dry eye syndrome

2. Blepharitis or meibomian gland dysfunction

3. Trachoma

4. Contact lens intolerance or overusage

5. Lacrimal infection: chronic dacryocystitis, chronic canaliculitis

6. Masquerading syndromes: intraepithelial neoplasia, malignant melanoma, sebaceous cell carcinoma

7. Superior limbic keratoconjunctivitis

8. Floppy eyelid syndrome

adherent to the underlying conjunctival tissue (**Figs. 9** and **10**). The underlying tissue can be friable when the membrane is gently removed with a sterile cotton applicator. This finding indicates a more severe inflammatory response.[9]

The examiner should strongly consider performing a Wood lamp examination with fluorescein staining to fully evaluate the cornea. Subtle findings such as herpes simplex virus (HSV) keratitis can be missed without this type of examination. HSV keratitis can present similarly to adenoviral conjunctivitis with watery discharge and absence of skin lesions. Fluorescein staining can reveal the classic corneal dendrites (**Fig. 2**).

Eyelid cultures and cytology should be obtained in cases of conjunctivitis that are resistant to treatment in infants and children and, in cases of hyperacute purulent conjunctivitis, in adults. In general, a topical anesthetic is not required when taking a sample from the skin or the exudates on the eyelids. If a conjunctival sample is indicated, a drop of proparacaine ophthalmic eye drop can be instilled for comfort. Rapid adenoviral testing is available to confirm the diagnosis of epidemic keratoconjunctivitis caused by adenovirus[10] (**Fig. 3**).

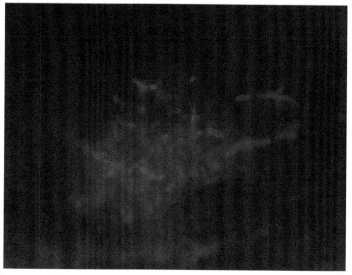

Fig. 2. HSV corneal dendrites stained with fluorescein and viewed under a Wood lamp. (*Courtesy of* Emory Eye Center, Emory University School of Medicine, Atlanta, GA.)

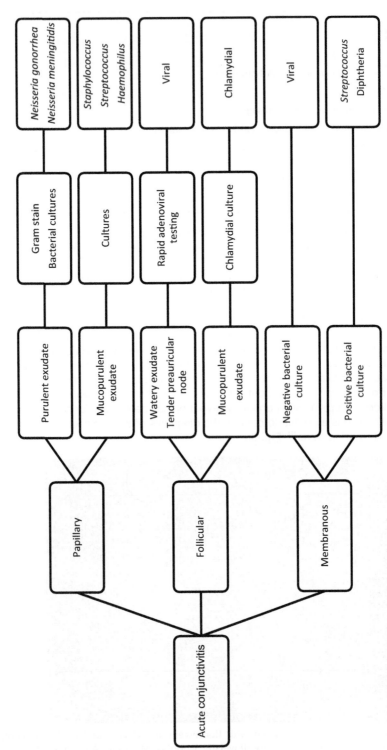

Fig. 3. Acute conjunctivitis. (*Adapted from* Buttross M, Stern GA. Acute conjunctivitis. In: Margo C, Hamed LM, Mames RN, editors. Diagnostic problems in clinical ophthalmology. Philadelphia: WB Saunders; 1994.)

CASE STUDY 1

A 9-month-old boy presents with a 2-day history of right eye redness. The mother states that the boy initially rubbed the eye profusely. She also notes increased yellowish discharge from the eye. The patient is otherwise healthy and up-to-date on his vaccinations. He recently started daycare.

Comments

This is a young child with a history of unilateral acute conjunctivitis.

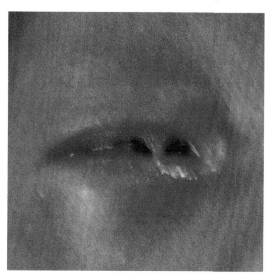

Fig. 4. Acute conjunctivitis of the right eye with mucopurulent discharge. (*Courtesy of Diana Shiba, MD, South Pasedena, CA.*)

On Examination

The boy appears to be able to fixate and follow objects with the right eye. The puslike discharge is adherent to the lashes but not copious (see **Fig. 4**). The periorbital area is slightly swollen and erythematous. It is difficult to determine whether there are papillary, follicular, or membranous changes on the conjunctiva because of the child's uncooperativeness.

Comments

The patient is presenting with mucopurulent discharge, which suggests a viral or bacterial cause that may include gonococcus, meningococcus, or chlamydia. It is important to obtain cultures of the skin and the exudate, but this can be performed without anesthetics and with minimal trauma.

Treatment

After obtaining cultures, initial treatment consisted of topical erythromycin ophthalmic eye ointment applied 4 times daily. After a few days, the culture tested positive for pan-sensitive *S aureus*.

Comments

Topical steroid or steroid combination drops should be avoided for several reasons in this case. Without the culture result, steroid eye drops can potentially worsen the infection. Topical steroids can have serious side effects that include glaucoma and cataract formation. The patient should be followed closely while on the appropriate antibiotic treatment. Periorbital cellulitis has been known to develop from conjunctivitis in young children. If there is any suspicion of periorbital cellulitis, the patient should be referred to ophthalmology emergently and treated with systemic antibiotics.

CASE STUDY 2

A 39-year-old woman presents with a 5-day history of a watery right eye (see **Fig. 5**). She has recently traveled on an airplane and is nursing a cold. She complains of progressively increasing watery discharge and itching. Otherwise, she is healthy.

Comments

This is a case of acute unilateral conjunctivitis.

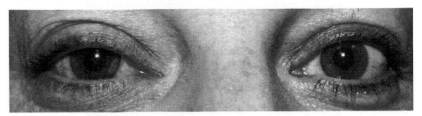

Fig. 5. Acute conjunctivitis of the right eye with watery discharge. (*Courtesy of* Emory Eye Center, Emory University School of Medicine, Atlanta, GA.)

On Examination

The patient's vision is normal. The palpebral conjunctiva shows evidence of follicular changes that are soft yellowish congregations of lymphoblasts (see **Fig. 6**). Follicles are usually easily seen in the lower palpebral conjunctiva.[9] The exudate appears watery. On palpation, she reports tenderness in the preauricular area.

Comments

The patient presents with classic symptoms and findings of viral conjunctivitis. The most common viral agent is adenovirus, which can also cause the common cold. The diagnosis can be confirmed with rapid adenoviral testing if needed.

Treatment

The patient prefers to treat her symptoms with conservative measures, which include cool compresses and chilled preservative-free artificial tears.

Comments

Patients with viral conjunctivitis should be educated on the contagious nature of the disease. They should practice frequent hand washing, avoid social activities, and avoid sharing personal items. The US Centers for Disease Control and Prevention recommends 2 weeks of patient contact avoidance for health care workers.[9] In most cases of viral conjunctivitis, topical steroids should be avoided because they can prolong viral replication and viral shedding. Misdiagnosis of HSV infection and superinfections are also of concern. However, topical nonsteroidal eye drops can be considered for comfort because they have no effect on viral replication or shedding. Antibiotic eye

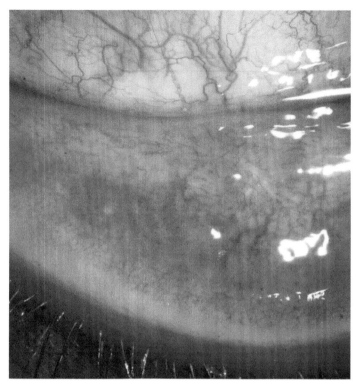

Fig. 6. Follicular changes on lower palpebral conjunctiva. (*Courtesy of* Emory Eye Center, Emory University School of Medicine, Atlanta, GA.)

drops are not indicated in viral conjunctivitis because secondary infection is a very rare occurrence.[9]

CASE STUDY 3

A 17-year-old white boy presents with a 2-week history of left eye redness. He was treated at an urgent care clinic 1 week ago with topical tobramycin eye drops, which did not improve his symptoms. He complains of redness, eye irritation, and discharge that sticks to the eye lashes.

Comments

The patient presents with acute unilateral conjunctivitis. His symptoms have not improved despite a course of antibiotic treatment. The differential diagnosis includes viral or atypical bacterial infections.

On Examination

The patient has normal vision. The patient has mucopurulent discharge from the left eye with no involvement of the right eye (**Fig. 7**). There appear to be follicles in the inferior conjunctiva (**Fig. 8**). Eyelid cultures are obtained to check for adenovirus, bacteria, and chlamydia. The results are positive for chlamydial antigens.

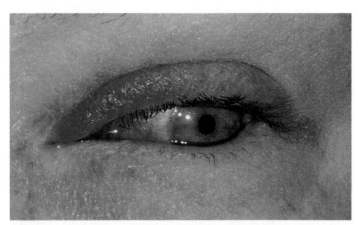

Fig. 7. Acute conjunctivitis of the left eye. (*Courtesy of* Emory Eye Center, Emory University School of Medicine, Atlanta, GA.)

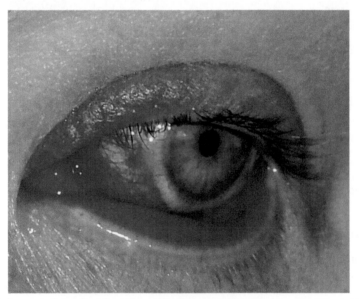

Fig. 8. Left eye inflamed conjunctiva. (*Courtesy of* Emory Eye Center, Emory University School of Medicine, Atlanta, GA.)

Comments

Inclusional or chlamydial conjunctivitis is unilateral and can self-resolve in 6 months. Eyelid cultures should be obtained in the case of unresolving conjunctivitis despite adequate treatment.

Treatment

The patient should be started on systemic oral antibiotics such as doxycycline for 1 to 2 weeks or 1 dose of azithromycin.

Comments

Chlamydial conjunctivitis should be considered a systemic disease requiring systemic treatment. Topical treatment is not necessary. The patient should be counseled regarding safe sex practices and the contagious nature of the disease. His sexual partners should also be examined and treated.

CASE STUDY 4

A 50-year-old female kindergarten teacher presents with a 5-day history of red eyes. The patient states that the redness began with the right eye then progressed to the left eye. She has had blurry vision in the last few days with increasing discharge and irritation. She had a recent episode of an upper respiratory infection. The symptoms have not improved with artificial tears.

Comments

This is a case of acute bilateral conjunctivitis. The cause could be viral, bacterial, or atypical bacterial.

On Examination

The patient has vision of 20/60 in both eyes. She has bilateral conjunctival membranes (see **Fig. 9**) and a tender right preauricular node. Membranes are inflammatory fibrin exudates attached to the underlying conjunctival epithelium (see **Fig. 10**). Eyelid cultures were taken. An appointment is scheduled with an ophthalmologist.

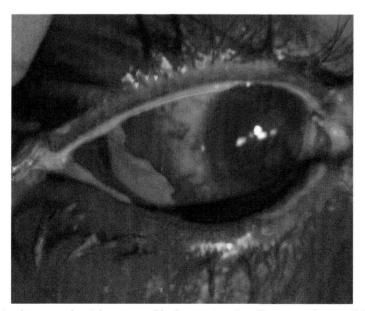

Fig. 9. Membrane on the right temporal bulbar conjunctiva. (*Courtesy of* Diana Shiba, MD, South Pasedena, CA.)

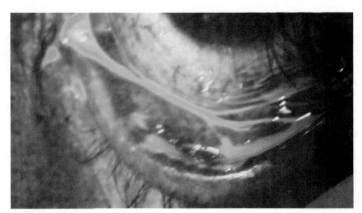

Fig. 10. Membrane on the inferior palpebral conjunctiva. (*Courtesy of* Diana Shiba, MD, South Pasedena, CA.)

Comments

Bilateral membranous conjunctivitis is a severe condition. The infectious agents could be viral, streptococcal, or diphtheria. A negative bacterial culture could indicate adenoviral infection. The sequelae can include severe conjunctival scarring and severe dry eyes. Prompt referral to ophthalmology is indicated.

CASE STUDY 5

A 40-year-old man presents with red and itchy eyes for more than 6 months. They usually have stringy clear discharge. He has been self-treating with over-the-counter vasoconstricting eye drops with no improvements.

Comments

This is a case of bilateral chronic conjunctivitis.

On Examination

The patient has normal vision. The conjunctiva is injected in both eyes. The upper eyelid was everted and showed multiple papillae (**Fig. 11**). Papillae are elevations in the conjunctiva with a central core of blood vessel usually found on the superior palpebral conjunctiva. They result from edema and polymorphonuclear cells infiltrating from the core vessel.[9]

Comments

Bilateral chronic papillary conjunctivitis usually indicates an allergic cause. In this patient's case, it is most likely atopic keratoconjunctivitis. It is important to make sure the patient is not a contact lens user because overusing contact lenses can present with a similar clinical picture. Atopic keratoconjunctivitis is different from vernal keratoconjunctivitis because the patients are usually older and the symptoms are independent of the seasons of the year (see **Fig. 12**).

Treatment

The patient is instructed to avoid known allergens and is educated on the benefits of frequent laundering of clothes and showering before bedtime. He was instructed to discontinue the use of over-the-counter vasoconstricting eye drops. These drops bring temporary relief, do not improve the inflammatory cause, and can be overused.

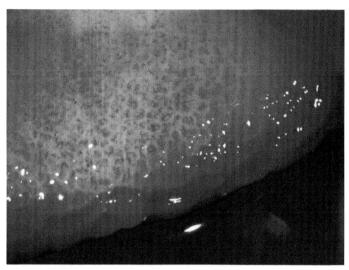

Fig. 11. Papillary changes on the upper palpebral conjunctiva. (*Courtesy of* Emory Eye Center, Emory University School of Medicine, Atlanta, GA.)

Initial treatment consists of a combination of preservative-free artificial tears, topical antihistamine, and topical mast cell stabilizers. Oral antihistamines can also be a part of the regimen. In some cases, a short course of topical steroids can be considered to improve symptoms. If topical steroids are indicated, the treatment should be initiated with the lowest potency and frequency. The patient should also be counseled on the potential side effects of topical steroids.[9]

Comments

A common comorbidity of chronic allergic conjunctivitis is dry eye syndrome. Oral antihistamines can exacerbate this condition. In some cases, long-term use of topical cyclosporine A provides antiinflammatory benefit for both dry eye and allergic components. In severe cases, it may be helpful to refer patients to an allergy specialist for allergen testing.

CASE STUDY 6

A 9-year-old African American boy presents with bilateral red eyes. His parents have noticed swelling and clear discharge from both eyes for about 1 month. The patient has been rubbing his eyes profusely and complaining of blurry vision. The patient also has a past medical history of atopic dermatitis and asthma.

Comments

The chronicity of the disease indicates that this is not an adenoviral infection; although common in this age group, these usually resolve in 10 days.

On Examination

The patient has decreased vision of 20/60 in the right eye and 20/30 in the left eye. The eyes are red with serous discharge and elevated limbal lesions (**Fig. 13**). With fluorescein staining, there appears to be a right corneal ulcer (**Fig. 14**). The patient was diagnosed with vernal keratoconjunctivitis and referred to an ophthalmologist urgently.

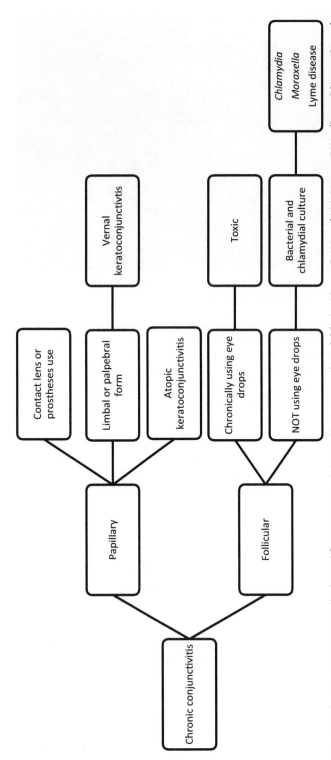

Fig. 12. Chronic conjunctivitis. (*Adapted from* Buttross M, Stern GA. Acute conjunctivitis. In: Margo C, Hamed LM, Mames RN, editors. Diagnostic problems in clinical ophthalmology. Philadelphia: WB Saunders; 1994.)

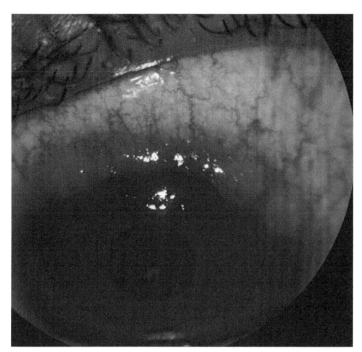

Fig. 13. Left eye limbal lesions in a patient with vernal conjunctivitis. (*Courtesy of* Emory Eye Center, Emory University School of Medicine, Atlanta, GA.)

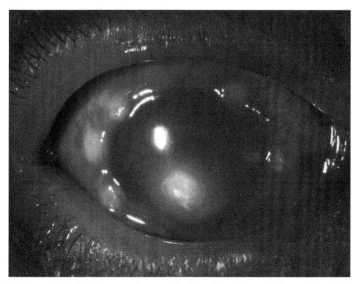

Fig. 14. Right eye limbal lesions and corneal ulcer. (*Courtesy of* Emory Eye Center, Emory University School of Medicine, Atlanta, GA.)

Comments

Vernal keratoconjunctivitis is usually found in young patients with presentation before the age of 10 years and usually resolution with the onset of puberty. There is a male predilection. Most patients have other systemic findings, such as asthma or eczema. The most common season of onset is spring, but symptoms can be present year-round. The finding of an ulcer on the peripheral cornea can be sight threatening.

Treatment

A patient with corneal findings should be referred to an ophthalmologist as soon as possible. Treatment involves avoidance of allergens, topical mast cell stabilizer drops, topical antihistamine drops, and oral antihistamine. In severe sight-threatening cases, topical and oral steroids can be used.

TREATMENT OF ALLERGIC CONJUNCTIVITIS

Treatment of allergic conjunctivitis begins with the avoidance of the causative allergen, if possible. Artificial tears serve to flush antigens and inflammatory mediators from the eyes as well as to provide a barrier. Pharmacologic agents used in the treatment of allergic conjunctivitis include antihistamines, multiple action antiallergic agents, and mast cell stabilizers. Antihistamines block histamine receptors, and relieve itching and redness, but only for a short time. However, these agents have no effect on other inflammatory mediators, such as prostaglandins and leukotrienes. Antihistamine decongestant combination agents may be more efficacious but are limited by short duration of action and need for dosing every 4 hours.[11] Mast cell stabilizers decrease degranulation of mast cells, which decreases histamine release and other chemotactic factors that are preformed or newly formed. These agents do not relieve existing symptoms. They can be used in advance of exposure to allergens to prevent mast cell degranulation, which may negatively affect medication adherence.

In general, mild symptoms should be treated with artificial tears and antihistamines. For symptoms that are more severe, persistent, or recurrent, these agents may be used in combination with decongestants and mast cell stabilizers.[10] More recently, multiple action drugs have been developed. These drugs work as H1 receptor antagonists by decreasing mast cell degranulation and by suppressing activation and infiltration of eosinophils. Examples of these are olopatadine, ketotifen, and azelastine.[12] Nonsteroidal antiinflammatory drugs also alleviate symptoms by decreasing pain and inflammation but are not as efficacious for allergic conjunctivitis as the dual-action agents.[12] Nonsteroidal medications are not associated with increased intraocular pressure or cataract formation, so they are preferred to steroidal medications. Corticosteroids decrease the inflammatory response associated with allergic conjunctivitis but are associated with risk of cataract formation and increased intraocular pressure. Two newer agents, loteprednol etabonate and difluprednate, seem to have improved side effect profiles compared with the older agents.[12] Immunomodulators are another class of drug used to treat allergic eye disease. These drugs act both by immunosuppression and immunostimulation. Two examples of these are cyclosporine A and tacrolimus. Cyclosporine A acts by decreasing eosinophil infiltration by limiting the type IV allergic response, and tacrolimus acts by decreasing the action of T cells. Both have been found to be effective and, in general, have few side effects and are preferred to ocular steroids in the treatment of allergic eye disease.[12] Immunomodulators attached to a more hydrophilic medium such as nanoparticles and other medications that show novel antiinflammatory effects are currently in development.[12] In general, steroids and immunomodulators should not be used in the primary care setting without ophthalmology consultation (**Table 2**).

Treatment of the severe forms of allergic conjunctival disease, such as AKC or VKC, usually involves the use of topical and oral antihistamines, ocular steroids, and cyclosporine. However, in cases of refractory disease, use of tacrolimus 0.1% has been shown to decrease total sign and symptom scores as well as giant papillae and corneal lesions.[13]

Subcutaneous immunotherapy (SCIT) and more recently sublingual immunotherapy (SLIT) are used to treat atopic disease such as conjunctivitis. The use of SLIT is currently considered off-label. A recent study concluded that the strength

Table 2
Ophthalmic agents for allergic conjunctivitis

Drug	Trade Name	Age, Dose	Cost ($)	Side Effects
H1-Antihistamines				
Emedastine difumarate	Emadine	≥3 y, 1 gtt qid	124	Headache 11%
Mast Cell Stabilizers				
Cromolyn	Opticrom and Crolom	≥2 y, 1–2 gtt qid	40	Burning, stinging, and itching <4%
Lodoxamide tromethamine	Alomide	≥2 y, 1–2 gtt qid	170	Burning, stinging, and itching 10%
Nedocromil	Alocril	≥3 y, 1–2 gtt bid	180	Headache, bitter taste, burning, and nasal congestion 10%
Pemirolast potassium	Alamast	≥3 y, 1–2 gtt qid	120	Burning, irritation, and nasal congestion <10%
H1-Antihistamines/Mast Cell Stabilizers Combination				
Alcaftadine	Lastacaft	≥3 y, 1–2 gtt q day	170	Burning, stinging, and itching <4%
Azelastine	Optivar	≥3 y, 1 gtt bid	105	Burning 10% Headache 15% Bitter taste 10%
Bepotastine	Bepreve	≥3 y, 1 gtt bid	300	Bitter taste 25% Headache, irritation, and nasopharyngitis 2%–5%
Epinastine	Elestat	≥3 y, 1 gtt bid	100	Cold symptoms 10%
Ketotifen	Zyrtec Eye and Claritin Eye	≥3 y, 1 gtt tid	20	Conjunctival injection, headache and rhinitis 10%–25%
Olopatadine	Pataday	≥3 y, 1–2 gtt q day	140	Headache 7%
Nonsteroidal Antiinflammatory Drugs				
Ketorolac tromethamine	Acular	≥12 y, 1 gtt qid	75	Burning, stinging, and itching 10%
Corticosteroid				
Loteprednol etabonate	Alrex	≥3 y, 1–2 gtt bid to qid	200	Headache, pharyngitis, and rhinitis 10%

Abbreviations: bid, two times a day; gtt, drops; q, every; qid, 4 times a day; tid, 3 times a day.

of evidence is low for SCIT and moderate for SLIT that either modality improved conjunctivitis symptoms.[14] Of the 2 regimens used to give immunotherapy, perennial immunotherapy (PIT) was associated with decreased symptom medication scores compared with preseason immunotherapy (PSIT). In PIT, an induction phase is followed by a maintenance phase that is continued until the treatment time is completed, whereas in PSIT the induction doses are given in sequential years before the allergy season.[15]

TREATMENT OF BACTERIAL CONJUNCTIVITIS

The distinction between acute (mucopurulent) bacterial and viral conjunctivitis on clinical findings can be difficult and, given that there is widespread belief among primary care providers that bacterial conjunctivitis requires treatment with antibiotics, most patients who are diagnosed in primary care practices receive topical antibiotics.[16] Previous data have suggested that acute bacterial conjunctivitis can be self-limited. Guidelines have been released in the United Kingdom to curb antibiotic use.[17] However, even in countries where guidelines exist and are accessible, antibiotic use remains high.[16] One potential treatment strategy is to identify those patients in whom antibiotic therapy might provide the most benefit. A patient data meta-analysis undertaken by Jefferis and colleagues[17] showed that age less than 5 years is the most sensitive predictor of a positive bacterial culture. The most specific predictor was age less than 5 years with moderate symptoms and purulent discharge. A Cochrane Review, updated in 2012 on the use of antibiotics for bacterial conjunctivitis, confirms that treatment with topical antibiotics hastens early resolution and offers a modest benefit on late resolution.[18] In addition, this review supports a delayed treatment strategy. Similar to strategies suggested for other infectious diseases, a delayed treatment strategy for acute bacterial conjunctivitis includes providing patient education on self-management techniques. Antibiotics are initiated if symptoms are not resolved in 3 days. This strategy was found by Everitt and colleagues[19] to be similar to providing immediate antibiotics and better than withholding antibiotics. We suggest written patient education on self-management strategies with consideration of the seasonality of the different types of conjunctivitis and, in the appropriate clinical setting, the prescription of topical antibiotics with an option to delay treatment for 2 to 3 days. In 2006, a Cochrane Review stated that patients treated with placebo have low risk of adverse events.[20] In addition, initiation of antibiotics may allow an earlier return to school, because several state departments of public health have guidelines prohibiting return to school until patients are treated with antibiotics.[21]

Hyperacute (purulent) conjunctivitis is commonly caused by *N gonorrhoeae* and *Pseudomonas aeruginosa* and is less commonly triggered by the microorganisms that cause acute conjunctivitis. This form of conjunctivitis is usually an effect of autoinoculation from infected genitalia and is most common during the warmer months.[22]

C trachomatis can cause 3 distinct types of ocular infection: neonatal conjunctivitis, adult inclusion conjunctivitis, and trachoma. Neonatal chlamydial conjunctivitis is transmitted from an infected mother during delivery and presents within the neonatal period with typical symptoms of conjunctivitis. The treatment is oral erythromycin base or ethyl succinate for 14 days. Antibiotic prophylaxis given during birth does not prevent chlamydial disease but is intended to prevent gonococcal infections.[23] Adult inclusion conjunctivitis is a mucopurulent conjunctivitis that is associated with concomitant genital disease and treated with oral doxycycline or erythromycin.[23] Trachoma is a chronic keratoconjunctivitis found mostly in sub-Saharan Africa. It occurs from recurrent infections with *C trachomatis* in children and leads to scarring, opacities, and blindness in adults. It is the most common cause of infectious blindness in the world.[24] The World Health Organization has established programs to eliminate trachoma through promotion of the SAFE strategy: surgery for trichiasis (eyelashes touching the eyeball), antibiotics, facial cleanliness, and environmental improvements. The antibiotics recommended are single doses of azithromycin or tetracycline ointment[24] (**Table 3**).

TREATMENT OF VIRAL CONJUNCTIVITIS

Viral conjunctivitis is an extremely common cause of conjunctivitis, with estimates as high as 80% of all causes of acute conjunctivitis.[6] As many as 90% of these cases of viral conjunctivitis are thought to be caused by human adenovirus, which is known to cause 2 distinct syndromes: epidemic keratoconjunctivitis and pharyngoconjunctival fever.[25] Pharyngoconjunctival fever classically presents as conjunctivitis, sore throat, fever, and preauricular lymphadenopathy. Epidemic keratoconjunctivitis is more severe and, as the name implies, can produce outbreaks in closed communities. In addition, this form of adenoviral ocular infection is associated with either formation of pseudomembranes or subepithelial infiltrates as complications.[25] Patients who experience complications should be referred to an ophthalmologist. Treatment is supportive and includes using cold compresses, artificial tears, careful attention to hand washing, and prevention of spread. This treatment encompasses isolation of patients with symptoms and exclusion of health care providers from patient care duties for 2 weeks.[25] In severe cases associated with complications, steroids and tacrolimus can be considered for use by an ophthalmologist.

Table 3
Ophthalmic agents for bacterial conjunctivitis

Drug	Trade Name	Dose	Cost ($)
Fluoroquinolones			
Besifloxacin 0.6%	Besivance	1 gtt tid × 7 d	160
Ciprofloxacin 0.3%	Ciloxan	1–2 gtt qid × 7 d	50
Levofloxacin 1.5%	Iquix	1–2 gtt qid × 7 d	88
Ofloxacin 0.3%	Ocuflox	1–2 gtt qid × 7 d	40
Levofloxacin 0.5%	Quixin	1–2 gtt qid × 7 d	75
Moxifloxacin 0.5%	Vigamox	1 gtt tid × 7 d	155
Gatifloxacin 0.3%	Zymar	1 gtt tid × 7 d	82
Aminoglycosides			
Tobramycin 0.3%	Tobrex	1–2 gtt qid × 7 d	20
Gentamicin 0.3%	Genoptic	1–2 gtt qid × 7 d	23
Polymyxin B Combinations			
Polymyxin B/trimethoprim	Polytrim	1 gtt q 4 h × 7–10 d	25
Polymyxin B/bacitracin	Polysporin	13 mm q 4 h × 7–10 d	30
Polymyxin B/neomycin/gramicidin	Neosporin	1–2 gtt q 4 h × 7–10 d	70
Other Antibiotics			
Azithromycin 1%	AzaSite	1 gtt q 12 h × 2 d then 1 gtt q day × 5 d	140
Erythromycin 0.5%	Ilotycin	13 mm q 4 h to q 12 h × 7 d	35

Adapted from Morrow GL, Abbott RL. Conjunctivitis. Am Fam Physician 1998;57(4):735–46.

An uncommon cause of conjunctivitis is herpes virus. However, both herpes simplex and herpes zoster virus can cause conjunctivitis. Herpes simplex can present as a unilateral red eye with vesicular eyelid lesions. This condition is treated with oral and topical antivirals, such as acyclovir. Herpes zoster can involve the eye, and a potential for ocular involvement must be assumed in the presence of lesions at the tip of the nose (Hutchinson sign). These patients should be referred to an ophthalmologist for full ophthalmic evaluation and treatment with oral antivirals.[6]

Prevention

Avoidance of the viral and bacterial contamination and known allergens is the key to conjunctivitis prevention. Frequent hand hygiene helps decrease the chances of disease transmission. Patients with bacterial and viral conjunctivitis should be counseled to minimize contacts, and to avoid returning to work or school and sharing personal items. Avoidance of known allergens is the key to prevent recurrence for most cases of allergic conjunctivitis. Patients should be instructed to stay indoors during high pollen counts, keep windows closed, shower frequently, wash hair before sleep, use mattress and pillow allergen covers, launder clothes and sheets frequently, avoid carpets, avoid pets, and minimize contact lens use.

SUMMARY

Conjunctivitis is the most common cause of red eye in primary care. The 3 most common types of conjunctivitis are viral, allergic, and bacterial, and they can present in either acute or chronic forms. The age of the patient, time of year, and physical examination findings are paramount to distinguish the different types of conjunctivitis. Nonetheless, distinguishing between acute viral and bacterial conjunctivitis remains difficult. Cases of allergic conjunctivitis should initially be treated with artificial tears and antihistamine or mast cell stabilizing drops. Viral conjunctivitis should also be treated conservatively with modalities such as artificial tears and cold compresses unless herpes simplex or zoster is suspected. These patients should be treated with topical and oral antivirals respectively and referred for ophthalmic evaluation. Antibiotics have been shown to improve symptoms in cases of acute bacterial conjunctivitis and may hasten return to school in some states. Adverse outcomes in cases of acute bacterial conjunctivitis, which are not treated with antibiotics, are very rare, and using a delayed treatment strategy before use of antibiotics may prevent unnecessary medication. Patients with prolonged symptoms, poor response to initial management, or evidence of severe disease should be referred to ophthalmology for consultation.

REFERENCES

1. Kaufman HE. Adenovirus advances: new diagnostic and therapeutic options. Curr Opin Ophthalmol 2011;22(4):290–3.
2. Shields T, Sloane PD. A comparison of eye problems in primary care and ophthalmology practices. Fam Med 1991;23(7):544–6.
3. Udeh BL, Schneider JE, Ohsfeldt RL. Cost effectiveness of a point-of-care test for adenoviral conjunctivitis. Am J Med Sci 2008;336(3):254–64.
4. Smith AF, Waycaster C. Estimate of the direct and indirect annual cost of bacterial conjunctivitis in the United States. BMC Ophthalmol 2009;9:13.
5. Thanathanee O, O'Brien TP. Conjunctivitis: systematic approach to diagnosis and therapy. Curr Infect Dis Rep 2011;13(2):141–8.
6. Azari AA, Barney NP. Conjunctivitis: a systematic review of diagnosis and treatment. JAMA 2013;310(16):1721–9.

7. Hovding G. Acute bacterial conjunctivitis. Acta Ophthalmol 2008;86(1):5–17.
8. Bielory BP, O'Brien TP, Bielory L. Management of seasonal allergic conjunctivitis: guide to therapy. Acta Ophthalmol 2012;90(5):399–407.
9. Krachmer JH, Holland EJ. Cornea. 2nd edition. Maryland Heights (MO): Mosby; 2005.
10. Association, T.E.M., <Preferred practice patterns from the AAO 2014.pdf>. American Academy of Ophthalmology, 2014.
11. La Rosa M, Lionetti E, Reibaldi M, et al. Allergic conjunctivitis: a comprehensive review of the literature. Ital J Pediatr 2013;39:18.
12. Mishra GP, Tamboli V, Jwala J, et al. Recent patents and emerging therapeutics in the treatment of allergic conjunctivitis. Recent Pat Inflamm Allergy Drug Discov 2011;5(1):26–36.
13. Fukushima A, Ohashi Y, Ebihara N, et al. Therapeutic effects of 0.1% tacrolimus eye drops for refractory allergic ocular diseases with proliferative lesion or corneal involvement. Br J Ophthalmol 2014;98(8):1023–7.
14. Kim JM, Lin SY, Suarez-Cuervo C, et al. Allergen-specific immunotherapy for pediatric asthma and rhinoconjunctivitis: a systematic review. Pediatrics 2013; 131(6):1155–67.
15. Tworek D, Bochenska-Marciniak M, Kuprys-Lipinska I, et al. Perennial is more effective than preseasonal subcutaneous immunotherapy in the treatment of seasonal allergic rhinoconjunctivitis. Am J Rhinol Allergy 2013;27(4):304–8.
16. Visscher KL, Hutnik CM, Thomas M. Evidence-based treatment of acute infective conjunctivitis: breaking the cycle of antibiotic prescribing. Can Fam Physician 2009;55(11):1071–5.
17. Jefferis J, Perera R, Everitt H, et al. Acute infective conjunctivitis in primary care: who needs antibiotics? An individual patient data meta-analysis. Br J Gen Pract 2011;61(590):e542–8.
18. Sheikh A, Hurwitz B, van Schayck CP, et al. Antibiotics versus placebo for acute bacterial conjunctivitis. Cochrane Database Syst Rev 2012;(9):CD001211.
19. Everitt HA, Little PS, Smith PW. A randomised controlled trial of management strategies for acute infective conjunctivitis in general practice. BMJ 2006;333(7563): 321.
20. Sheikh A, Hurwitz B. Antibiotics versus placebo for acute bacterial conjunctivitis. Cochrane Database Syst Rev 2006;(2):CD001211.
21. Ohnsman CM. Exclusion of students with conjunctivitis from school: policies of state departments of health. J Pediatr Ophthalmol Strabismus 2007;44(2):101–5.
22. Quinn CJ, Mathews DE, Noyes RF, et al. Optometric clinical practice guideline care of the patient with conjunctivitis. St. Louis, MO: American Optometric Association; 2002. p. 33.
23. Mishori R, McClaskey EL, WinklerPrins VJ. *Chlamydia trachomatis* infections: screening, diagnosis, and management. Am Fam Physician 2012;86(12): 1127–32.
24. Hu VH, Harding-Esch EM, Burton MJ, et al. Epidemiology and control of trachoma: systematic review. Trop Med Int Health 2010;15(6):673–91.
25. Gonzalez-Lopez JJ, Morcillo-Laiz R, Munoz-Negrete FJ. Adenoviral keratoconjunctivitis: an update. Arch Soc Esp Oftalmol 2013;88(3):108–15.

Acute Vision Loss

Nika Bagheri, MD[a], Sonia Mehta, MD[b],*

KEYWORDS

- Amaurosis fugax • Vertebrobasilar insufficiency • Migraine • Vitreous hemorrhage
- Retinal detachment • Retinal vascular occlusion • Papilledema • Optic neuritis
- Ischemic optic neuropathy

KEY POINTS

- When a patient presents with acute vision loss, it is important to determine the duration of vision loss and if it has affected one eye or both eyes.
- Transient causes of acute vision loss, lasting less than 24 hours, include amaurosis fugax, vertebrobasilar artery insufficiency, and migraine.
- Common causes of acute vision loss lasting greater than 24 hours include acute angle closure glaucoma, vitreous hemorrhage, retinal detachment, retinal artery occlusion, retinal vein occlusion, optic neuritis, ischemic optic neuropathy, and cerebrovascular accident.
- Patients complaining of acute vision loss with additional neurologic symptoms such as weakness, numbness, paresthesia, dysarthria, dysphagia, or headache should be sent to the emergency room immediately.
- Patients with acute vision loss without neurologic symptoms should be referred to ophthalmology immediately to determine the cause of the vision loss.

ACUTE VISION LOSS

Causes of acute vision loss are described in **Table 1**. Acute vision loss can be transient (lasting <24 hours) or persistent (lasting >24 hours). When evaluating a patient with acute vision loss, it is important to determine whether the vision loss affected one eye or both eyes.

TRANSIENT VISION LOSS
Amaurosis Fugax

Amaurosis fugax is monocular transient vision loss due to lack of blood flow and perfusion to the optic nerve and retina. It is painless, and patients classically describe a dark curtain

Financial Disclosure: The authors have no financial interest on the devices or medications in this document. The authors have no conflicts of interest.
[a] Wills Eye Hospital, Department of Ophthalmology, Thomas Jefferson University, 840 Walnut Street, Suite 800, Philadelphia, PA 19107, USA; [b] Vitreoretinal Diseases & Surgery Service, Wills Eye Hospital, Department of Ophthalmology, Thomas Jefferson University Hospital, 840 Walnut Street, Suite 1020, Philadelphia, PA 19107, USA
* Corresponding author.
E-mail address: soniamehtamd@gmail.com

Prim Care Clin Office Pract 42 (2015) 347–361
http://dx.doi.org/10.1016/j.pop.2015.05.010
0095-4543/15/$ – see front matter © 2015 Elsevier Inc. All rights reserved.

primarycare.theclinics.com

Table 1 Causes of acute vision loss	
Transient Vision Loss	**Persistent Vision Loss**
Unilateral	
Amaurosis fugax	Acute angle closure glaucoma
	Vitreous hemorrhage
	Retinal detachment
	Retinal artery occlusion
	Retinal vein occlusion
	Optic neuritis
	Ischemic optic neuropathy
Bilateral	
Papilledema	Cerebrovascular accident
Vertebrobasilar artery insufficiency	
Migraine	

or shade coming over their vision. Causes include carotid artery disease, other atherosclerotic disease, embolic disease from the heart or aorta, hypercoagulable/hyperviscosity state, illicit drugs such as cocaine, and rarely inflammation of the arteries.

Symptom criteria

- Painless, monocular vision loss with resolution of symptoms after seconds to minutes
- Darkening of vision
- May have presyncopal symptoms

Clinical findings

Physical examination typically shows age-appropriate ophthalmic findings with normal visual acuity, pupillary responses, and color vision. A dilated fundus examination may show signs of chronic underlying ischemic disease (ie, hypertension, diabetes) with arteriovenous nicking, attenuated vessels, cotton wool spots, or retinal hemorrhages.

Diagnostic modalities

Amaurosis fugax is a classic symptom of carotid artery disease. Workup must evaluate for sources of emboli and ischemia, including imaging with bilateral carotid Doppler ultrasonography and/or magnetic resonance angiography (MRA)/computed tomography (CT) angiography of the neck and/or head. An echocardiogram may be indicated to evaluate for embolic heart disease. Basic laboratory tests evaluating risk factors for hematologic and atherosclerotic disease, such as complete blood count (CBC), fasting blood glucose or hemoglobin A1C levels, and cholesterol levels, should be done to rule out other causes of ischemia and to optimize health maintenance.

Management goals

Prompt evaluation and workup is indicated to determine the extent of underlying systemic disease and to address risk factors for stroke. Modifiable risk factors, especially smoking, should be addressed, and the patient strongly advised to quit.[1] For symptomatic carotid artery disease with evidence of greater than 70% ipsilateral stenosis, carotid endarterectomy is indicated and reduces the risk of stroke by 70%.[2,3] In cases with less than 70% ipsilateral stenosis, long-term aspirin administration (325 mg) is indicated.[2,3]

Referral strategies
Patients with amarousis fugax should be sent to an emergency room for prompt vascular imaging to determine the extent of underlying disease. These patients have high risk for stroke.

Self-management strategies
Patients with amarousis fugax should have their modifiable risk factors optimized and undergo a thorough evaluation for blood pressure, blood sugar, and serum cholesterol as well as smoking cessation.

Comanagement goals: evaluation, adjustment, recurrence
Patients with amarousis fugax who are candidates should be referred to a vascular surgeon for carotid endarterectomy. Patients should be evaluated by an ophthalmologist to determine if there are other findings that support a cause for vision loss. Addressing the systemic disease significantly improves the patient's long-term morbidity and mortality.

Summary
Amaurosis fugax is characterized by monocular, transient vision loss due to decreased blood perfusion of the optic nerve and retina. It is classically associated with carotid artery disease but can also occur due to emboli from other sources, a hypercoagulable state, arteritis, and recreational drug use. Once the condition is suspected, the patient should be sent to the emergency room for vascular imaging and workup of ischemic disease. Patients who are found to have carotid occlusive disease have significant improvement in morbidity and mortality by preventing stroke once appropriately managed.

Papilledema

Papilledema is bilateral optic disc swelling secondary to elevated intracranial pressure. It typically causes transient bilateral vision loss lasting a few seconds. Patients typically note the vision changes when changing positions, such as from supine to standing. Causes include primary or metastatic intracranial tumor, intracranial hemorrhage, malformation, obstructive hydrocephalus (decreases cerebrospinal fluid [CSF] drainage), brain abscess, meningitis, encephalitis, venous sinus thrombosis, venous outflow obstruction, idiopathic intracranial hypertension (IIH) (pseudotumor cerebri), choroid plexus tumor (increased CSF production), or craniosynostosis (decreased skull volume).

Symptom criteria
Patients with papilledema may experience the following:

- Transient vision loss lasting seconds and precipitated by postural changes
- Headache
- Nausea
- Vomiting
- Pulsatile tinnitus
- Double vision

Clinical findings
Visual acuity, color vision, and pupillary responses in patients with papilledema can be normal. Visual field testing in patients with bilateral papilledema may reveal an enlarged blind spot. On fundus examination, patients have bilateral optic disc swelling (**Fig. 1**), in which the disc margins appear blurred and the optic nerve is elevated. In

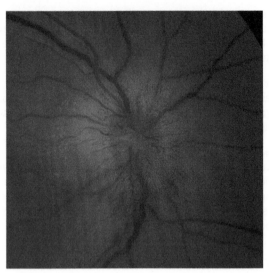

Fig. 1. Optic disc swelling in a patient with papilledema. Note that the disc margins appear blurred.

addition, patients can have retinal hemorrhages overlying or adjacent to the optic nerve.

Diagnostic modalities

Blood pressure should be checked because optic nerve swelling can occur in malignant hypertension. MRI with gadolinium and magnetic resonance venography of the head and orbits should be performed. CT scan should be done if MRI is not readily available. If the neuroimaging does not reveal an intracranial mass or hydrocephalus, lumbar puncture with CSF analysis and opening pressure measurement should be done. The purpose of the diagnostic testing is to confirm the diagnosis of papilledema and also to help determine the underlying cause.

Management goals

The cause of the papilledema should be determined and addressed. In patients with IIH, acetazolamide is recommended. This drug can help with headaches and vision loss.[4] Patients should be asked about medications, including birth control and tetracyclines, as these can exacerbate or precipitate IIH. In addition, weight loss is important, as it can help to reverse vision problems from the disease.[4,5] In patients with progressive vision loss despite treatment with acetazolamide, optic nerve sheath fenestration can be performed to help relieve pressure around the optic nerve surgically.[6] In those patients with progressive vision problems and severe headaches not improving on medical therapy, neurosurgical consultation is recommended for evaluation of shunt placement.[7]

Referral strategies

Patients with papilledema should be sent to the emergency room for neuroimaging and/or lumbar puncture to determine the cause of the increased intracranial pressure.

Self-management strategies

IIH tends to occur in young overweight women. In this condition, weight loss is helpful in preventing additional vision loss and also reversing vision loss from the disease.

Comanagement goals: evaluation, adjustment, recurrence
Patients with papilledema should have an examination by an ophthalmologist to determine the extent of their vision loss. Papilledema when left untreated can result in progressive and permanent vision loss over time. More severe vision loss requires more frequent follow-up. If the underlying cause of the intracranial hypertension is not addressed, then this can result in severe morbidity and mortality.

Summary
Papilledema is optic disc swelling from increased intracranial hypertension and can occur in conditions such as intracranial tumors, intracranial hemorrhages, infections, venous sinus thrombosis, and hydrocephalus. Once diagnosed, the patient should be sent to the emergency room for neuroimaging and/or lumbar puncture to determine the cause of the increased intracranial pressure and for treatment. If left untreated, papilledema can result in progressive, permanent vision loss over time. Furthermore, significant morbidity and mortality may occur from the underlying condition.

Vertebrobasilar Insufficiency

Vertebrobasilar insufficiency causes transient bilateral vision loss secondary to decreased ocular perfusion. Vision loss lasts seconds and may be accompanied by photopsias as well as neurologic symptoms such as dysarthria, vertigo, focal weakness, or numbness. Causes include embolic disease, other atherosclerotic disease, hypercoagulable/hyperviscosity states, and rarely vasculitis.

Symptom criteria

- Transient bilateral vision loss lasting a few seconds, often recurrent
- Dysarthria
- Ataxia
- Focal weakness or numbness

Clinical findings
The ophthalmic examination findings are within normal limits with normal pupillary responses and color vision. A dilated fundus examination may show signs of chronic ischemic disease (ie, hypertension, diabetes) with arteriovenous nicking, attenuated vessels, cotton wool spots, or retinal hemorrhages.

Diagnostic modalities
Vertebrobasilar insufficiency requires a comprehensive vascular and ischemic workup, including neuroimaging such as MRI and MRA to evaluate posterior blood flow, carotid Doppler ultrasonography, and echocardiography. Blood pressure should be checked in both arms. Basic laboratory tests evaluating risk factors for hematologic and atherosclerotic disease, such as CBC, fasting blood glucose or hemoglobin A1C levels, and cholesterol levels, should be done to optimize health maintenance.

Management goals
Prompt evaluation and workup is indicated to determine the extent of underlying systemic disease and to address risk factors for stroke. Select patients may require a referral to an endovascular surgeon or interventionalist for surgical correction.[8–10]

Referral strategies
Patients with vertebrobasilar insufficiency should be sent to an emergency room for prompt neurovascular imaging to determine the extent of underlying disease. These patients are at high risk for stroke.

Self-management strategies

Patients with vertebrobasilar insufficiency should have their modifiable risk factors optimized and undergo a thorough evaluation for blood pressure, blood sugar, and serum cholesterol, as well as smoking cessation counseling.

Comanagement goals: evaluation, adjustment, recurrence

Patients should be evaluated by an ophthalmologist, with a dilated fundus examination that may show retinal emboli or optic nerve changes. If there is any concern by history or ophthalmic finding for giant cell arteritis, emergent treatment is indicated.

Summary

Vertebrobasilar insufficiency may cause bilateral, transient vision loss as a result of decreased posterior cerebral blood flow. It often may recur and occur in conjunction with strokelike symptoms, such as dysarthria, ataxia, and focal weakness or numbness. Patients with vertebrobasilar insufficiency have high long-term morbidity and mortality, and optimizing control of their risk factors is urgent.

Migraine

Please see article.[11]

PERSISTENT VISION LOSS

Vitreous Hemorrhage

Please see article.[11]

Retinal Detachment

Please see article.[11]

Retinal Artery Occlusion

Occlusion of a branch or the central retinal artery causes unilateral, painless vision loss due to decreased retinal perfusion that ranges in severity from partial field loss to profound loss of vision. Causes include embolic or atherosclerotic disease, thrombosis and/or hypercoagulable state, inflammation of arteries (ie, giant cell arteritis), and less commonly collagen vascular disease.

Symptom criteria

- Painless, unilateral vision loss
- May have history of amaurosis fugax symptoms

Clinical findings

Ophthalmic examination shows whitening of the retina along the distribution of the retinal artery (**Fig. 2**). Patients may have an afferent pupillary defect, a cherry-red spot in the macula with central retinal artery occlusion, and the fundus may show cotton wool spots or cholesterol emboli (Hollenhorst plaque).

Diagnostic modalities

Blood pressure should be checked and basic laboratory tests should be performed to rule out malignant hypertension or coagulation disorder. Carotid Doppler ultrasonography and echocardiography are performed to search for emboli. If a Hollenhorst plaque is visualized, patient should undergo additional neuroimaging.

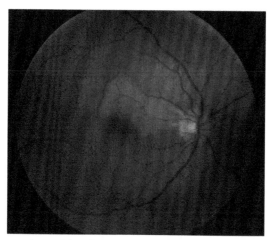

Fig. 2. Fundus in a patient with a branch retinal artery occlusion. Note the presence of retinal whitening corresponding to ischemia in the distribution of the blocked artery.

Management goals

Identifying the cause for the retinal artery occlusion is the primary goal. An embolic workup including carotid Doppler ultrasonography and echocardiography should be performed.[12] If there is suspicion for giant cell arteritis in a patient with central retinal artery occlusion, appropriate tests are warranted and the patient should be emergently administered high-dose intravenous corticosteroids.[13] A retinal artery occlusion in a young patient warrants a comprehensive assessment for hypercoagulable states and collagen vascular diseases.[14] If a Hollenhorst plaque is visualized, the patient should be admitted for stroke workup.

Referral strategies

Patients with a retinal artery occlusion should be referred to the emergency room for prompt embolic workup.

Self-management strategies

The most common cause of retinal artery occlusion is atherosclerotic disease with emboli. Patients with this condition benefit from comprehensive evaluation and modification of risk factors (blood pressure, blood sugar, serum cholesterol, and smoking cessation counseling).

Comanagement goals: evaluation, adjustment, recurrence

Patients should be evaluated by an ophthalmologist with a dilated fundus examination to evaluate for signs of ischemia and emboli. A fluorescein angiogram may be performed in the office setting to confirm the diagnosis.

Summary

Retinal artery occlusion causes unilateral permanent vision loss of varying severity. Patients with this condition warrant an embolic workup and risk factor modification for hypertension, diabetes, hyperlipidemia, and smoking cessation. Care should be taken to rule out giant cell arteritis in patients at risk who present with central retinal artery occlusion. Any young patient with retinal artery occlusion should undergo a comprehensive evaluation for underlying hypercoagulable disease or collagen vascular disease.

Retinal Vein Occlusion

Occlusion of a branch or the central retinal vein causes unilateral, painless vision loss secondary to venous stasis causing edema, hemorrhage, and possible ischemia. Loss of vision ranges in severity from partial field loss to profound loss of vision. Causes include compression from adjacent retinal arteries due to atherosclerotic disease (eg, hypertension, diabetes), hypercoagulable state, and rarely collagen vascular disease.[15,16] Glaucoma is also a risk factor.[15,16]

Symptom criteria

- Painless, unilateral vision loss

Clinical findings

Ophthalmic examination shows variable visual acuity deficit depending on the location of the branch vein or if central vein occlusion. A dilated fundus examination shows large-caliber tortuous vessels with edema along distribution of the affected retinal vein (**Fig. 3**). The classic blood and thunder fundus with hemorrhages and dilated vessels in all 4 quadrants occurs in central vein occlusion (**Fig. 4**).

Diagnostic modalities

Blood pressure should be checked and basic laboratory tests done. Further laboratory workup for less common causes is indicated based on history and review of systems.

Management goals

Typical retinal vein occlusion does not require the same emergent embolic workup as for retinal artery occlusion, because the cause is compression from chronic atherosclerotic disease. In cases in which the patient does not have risk factors such as hypertension or diabetes, or if the patient is young, it is important to conduct further laboratory workup for inflammatory or hematologic causes.[17]

Referral strategies

Patients with retinal vein occlusion due to underlying hematologic or collagen vascular disease should be referred for evaluation by a hematologist or rheumatologist, respectively. Retinal vein occlusion conveys an increased cardiovascular risk and may require cardiology referral for management of risk factors.[18]

Self-management strategies

Most of the retinal vein occlusion is secondary to chronic atherosclerotic disease. Patients with this condition benefit from comprehensive evaluation and modification of risk factors, the most important of which is hypertension.

Comanagement goals: evaluation, adjustment, recurrence

Patients should be evaluated by an ophthalmologist with a dilated fundus examination to evaluate for signs of ischemia and emboli. A fluorescein angiogram may be performed in the office setting to determine the amount of associated ischemia (see **Fig. 3**B), and patients require surveillance to monitor for possible development of neovascular disease, macular edema (see **Fig. 3**C), or glaucoma. Patients may require sequential intravitreal injections for treatment of associated macular edema.

Summary

Retinal vein occlusion causes unilateral permanent vision loss of varying severity. These occlusions typically occur as a result of chronic atherosclerotic disease, and patients require management of risk factors, including hypertension, diabetes, hyperlipidemia, and smoking cessation. Care should be taken to order a hypercoagulability

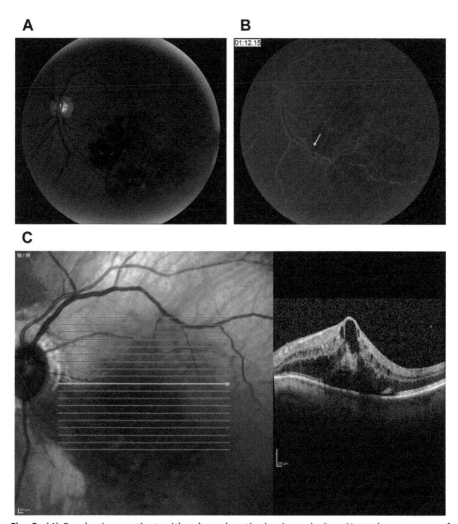

Fig. 3. (*A*) Fundus in a patient with a branch retinal vein occlusion. Note the presence of intraretinal hemorrhages and cotton wool spots along the obstructed retinal vein. (*B*) A fluorescein angiogram was performed demonstrating the site of blockage (*arrow*). (*C*) Optical coherence tomography of the macula demonstrated the presence of severe macular edema.

panel and evaluate for collagen vascular disease in patients who do not have the classic risk factors or who have concerning history or review of systems.

Optic Neuritis

Optic neuritis is inflammation of the optic nerve resulting in progressive loss of vision over the course of days. It is typically unilateral, associated with pain (especially with eye movements), and more often occurs in young to middle-aged women. It can be associated with systemic demyelinating disease. Causes include demyelinating disease (eg, multiple sclerosis), infection (eg, syphilis, Lyme disease, viral infection), and granulomatous disease (eg, sarcoidosis).

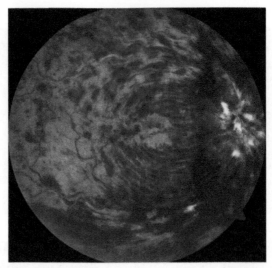

Fig. 4. Fundus in a patient with a central retinal vein occlusion. Note the blood and thunder appearance from the multiple intraretinal hemorrhages and dilated and tortuous vessels.

Symptom criteria

- Progressive vision loss typically over the course of days
- Reduced perception of light intensity and color brightness
- Pain with extraocular movements
- May have neurologic symptoms such as weakness or tingling

Clinical findings

Ophthalmic examination may show a relative afferent pupillary defect, decreased color vision, central or cecocentral scotoma, and optic nerve head edema in about a third of patients.

Diagnostic modalities

All first episodes or atypical cases should be evaluated with an MRI of the brain and orbits with gadolinium to confirm enhancement of the involved optic nerve and to assess for signs of intracranial pathology. In atypical cases, laboratory tests including CBC, erythrocyte sedimentation rate (ESR), ACE, Lyme antibodies, and RPR/FTA-Abs may be considered. Rare cases may require lumbar puncture.

Management goals

First episodes of optic neuritis warrant neuroimaging. If demyelinating disease is detected, patients should be treated with intravenous corticosteroids and referred to a neurologist.[19,20] Intravenous steroids improve the rapidity of visual recovery, although they do not affect final visual acuity outcomes.[19,20] If laboratory testing reveals abnormalities, further workup and treatment of the underlying disease (eg, syphilis) is indicated.[21]

Referral strategies

Patients with optic neuritis should be sent to the emergency room for neuroimaging (MRI brain/orbits with gadolinium) and possible admission for administration of intravenous corticosteroids.

Self-management strategies
Untreated optic neuritis typically improves without treatment, although visual recovery may be incomplete and take several weeks.

Comanagement goals: evaluation, adjustment, recurrence
Patients with optic neuritis and evidence of demyelinating disease (ie, multiple sclerosis) on neuroimaging should be referred to a neurologist for consideration of early initiation of therapy for multiple sclerosis. The patient should also be followed up by an ophthalmologist to determine the extent of visual deficit and recovery and to conduct visual field testing.

Summary
Optic neuritis is inflammation of the optic nerve causing progressive, painful visual loss. It may be associated with neurologic symptoms such as focal weakness or numbness and is a common initial manifestation of multiple sclerosis. Optic neuritis may also occur because of systemic inflammatory disease (eg, sarcoidosis) as well as infectious causes. Patients require neuroimaging to confirm the diagnosis as optic nerve edema is not present on examination most of the time. Patients may require intravenous steroids and comanagement with neurology and ophthalmology to monitor and treat visual field loss. Visual prognosis is variable but correlates to vision at presentation.

Ischemic Optic Neuropathy

Ischemic optic neuropathy occurs secondary to low perfusion and may involve the anterior or posterior portion of the optic nerve. A distinguishing feature of optic neuritis includes painless, sudden vision loss typically occurring in older patients with vascular risk factors. Anterior ischemic optic neuropathy is idiopathic but associated with many risk factors and abnormal autoregulation of normal optic nerve flow and nocturnal hypotension. Risk factors include atherosclerotic disease, hypertension (and the use of antihypertensive medication before sleeping), smoking, diabetes, sleep apnea, and medications such as amiodarone and phosphodiesterase inhibitors. Giant cell arteritis is a distinct entity that causes inflammation and obstruction of blood flow leading to anterior optic neuropathy. Posterior ischemic optic neuropathy (PION) occurs because of decreased blood flow due to intraoperative hypotension, anemia, or high-risk head positioning (Trendelenburg position). It classically occurs in patients who have experienced lengthy abdominal/cardiothoracic/spine procedures. A history of atherosclerosis can make patients more susceptible to PION.

Symptom criteria

- Painless vision loss, typically unilateral in anterior cases, may be bilateral in posterior cases
- Altitudinal visual field defect
- Reduced color vision
- Patients with giant cell arteritis may have typical symptoms including jaw claudication, headache, weight loss, fever, or proximal muscle ache (polymyalgia rheumatica)

Clinical findings
Ophthalmic examination may show a relative afferent pupillary defect, color plate deficit, moderate to significant visual field loss, and optic disc swelling with or without hemorrhages. There is a range of possibilities for optic nerve head appearance. Patients with giant cell arteritis may have a pale chalky white, swollen nerve. Patients

with posterior ischemic optic neuropathies may initially have normal-appearing optic nerves. Optic nerve pallor suggests old ischemia.

Diagnostic modalities
Vital signs, including blood pressure, should be measured. All patients older than 55 years with risk factors should have a CBC/ESR/c-reactive protein drawn to assess for giant cell arteritis. If the index of suspicion for giant cell arteritis is sufficiently high, a temporal artery biopsy is indicated regardless of laboratory results. In the absence of typical atherosclerotic risk factors, MRI of the orbits with gadolinium should be considered.

Management goals
Giant cell arteritis must be ruled out early on, as there is a substantial risk of early involvement of the contralateral eye and permanent bilateral visual impairment. If the index of suspicion for giant cell arteritis is high, immediate intravenous high-dose corticosteroids and scheduling of temporal artery biopsy should be considered.[22] In all other cases, there is no proven therapy to change final visual outcome, although there are reports of improvement with systemic corticosteroids.[23,24] Goals are to minimize associated risk factors such as hypertension, diabetes, sleep apnea, and medications. Primary care physicians should consider moving nighttime blood pressure medications to the morning to avoid nocturnal hypotension.[25]

Referral strategies
Patients with ischemic optic neuropathy should be sent to the emergency room for prompt evaluation by an ophthalmologist, laboratory testing to rule out giant cell arteritis, and possible admission for intravenous corticosteroids. Patients with suspected sleep apnea on history should be referred for a formal sleep study.

Self-management strategies
For patients with giant cell arteritis requiring long-term corticosteroids, blood pressure and blood sugar should be monitored in addition to bone density measurements to assess for osteoporotic changes. In all other cases, management of hypertension, diabetes, and other systemic risk factors through lifestyle modifications may reduce the risk of future ischemic events. Patients with sleep apnea should use a continuous positive airway pressure machine.

Comanagement goals: evaluation, adjustment, recurrence
Patients with ischemic optic neuropathy should have an examination and follow-up by an ophthalmologist to determine the extent and recovery of their vision loss. In cases of giant cell arteritis, referral to rheumatology should be considered for monitoring of corticosteroid therapy.

Summary
Ischemic optic neuropathy causes painless, sudden vision loss. Regardless of cause treatment focuses on reducing risk of further visual impairment through risk factor reduction. Giant cell arteritis must always be considered in the appropriate age group and setting given the efficacy of corticosteroid treatment and the potential consequences of delayed treatment. In other cases of suspected nocturnal hypotension, the timing of antihypertensive medications should be investigated and changed if possible to avoid nocturnal hypotension.

Cerebrovascular Accident

Cerebrovascular accident, or stroke, results from disturbance of cerebral perfusion, with resultant infarction leading to functional deficit. Visual impairment can range from none to severe depending on the location and extent of infarction. Strokes may be ischemic, embolic (eg, carotid atherosclerotic disease), or hemorrhagic (eg, subarachnoid hemorrhage) and may be precipitated by underlying risk factors such as smoking and rarely infectious or inflammatory causes.

Symptom criteria

- Focal weakness
- Numbness
- Dysarthria
- Aphasia
- Dysphagia
- Visual field deficits
- Headache

Clinical findings

Physical examination shows focal neurologic deficits such as weakness, loss of sensation, dysarthria, and aphasia. Ophthalmic examination shows normal pupillary responses, but patients may have visual field loss, including homonymous hemianopsia or quadrantanopsia. Dilated fundus examination would be unremarkable in terms of optic nerve and fundus appearance.

Diagnostic modalities

Any patient with a suspected cerebrovascular accident needs stat transport to the nearest emergency room facility for initiation of stroke protocol. Patients should undergo neuroimaging with CT and MRI to evaluate for hemorrhagic versus ischemic or embolic strokes.

Management goals

Initial management in the emergency room consists of time-sensitive evaluation and treatment of vital signs to reduce mortality and morbidity.[26,27] Pharmacologic therapy should be initiated promptly as per stroke protocol. Visual evaluation should take secondary precedence to life-sustaining measures.

Referral strategies

Once patients are emergently stabilized, inpatient ophthalmology consultation should be considered for evaluation of visual complaints including visual field deficits. Patients should be followed up by a neurologist and may need a cardiology referral depending on risk factors.

Self-management strategies

Life-style modifications are critical to prevent future vascular events such as recurrent cerebrovascular accident or myocardial infarction. Visual impairment may preclude patients from driving and they may need assistance with activities of daily living.

Comanagement goals: evaluation, adjustment, recurrence

Outpatient ophthalmology follow-up may be warranted to document severity with formal visual fields. Patients require long-term neurology follow-up and may benefit from physical, occupational, or speech therapy depending on deficits.

Summary

Cerebrovascular accident is a devastating and potentially life-threatening entity that represents the third leading cause of death in the United States. Visual deficits may occur and range in severity depending on the location of infarction. Once stabilized, patients may ultimately benefit from a multidisciplinary approach for rehabilitation.

REFERENCES

1. Biller J, Feinberg WM, Castaldo JE, et al. Guidelines for carotid endarterectomy: a statement for healthcare professionals from a Special Writing Group of the Stroke Council, American Heart Association. Circulation 1998;97:501–9.
2. North American Symptomatic Carotid Endarterectomy Trial (NASCET) study investigators. Clinical alert: benefit of carotid endarterectomy for patients with high-grade stenosis of the internal carotid artery. National Institute of Neurological Disorders and Stroke and Trauma Division. Stroke 1991;22:816–7.
3. ECST study investigators. Randomized trial of endarterectomy for recently symptomatic carotid stenosis: final results of the MRC European Carotid Surgery Trial (ECST). Lancet 1998;351:1379–87.
4. NORDIC Idiopathic Intracranial Hypertension Study Group Writing Committee, Wall M, McDermott MP, et al. Effect of acetazolamide on visual function in patients with idiopathic intracranial hypertension and visual loss: the idiopathic intracranial hypertension treatment trial. JAMA 2014;311:1641–51.
5. Banik R. Obesity and the role of nonsurgical and surgical weight reduction in idiopathic intracranial hypertension. Int Ophthalmol Clin 2014;54:27–41.
6. Alsuhaibani AH, Carter KD, Nerad JA, et al. Effect of optic nerve sheath fenestration on papilledema of the operated and the contralateral nonoperated eyes in idiopathic intracranial hypertension. Ophthalmology 2011;118:412–4.
7. Mukherjee N, Bhatti MT. Update on the surgical management of idiopathic intracranial hypertension. Curr Neurol Neurosci Rep 2014;14:438.
8. Shutze W, Gierman J, McQuade K, et al. Treatment of proximal vertebral artery disease. Vascular 2014;22:85–92.
9. Mokin M, Dumont TM, Kass-Hout T, et al. Carotid and vertebral artery disease. Prim Care 2013;40:135–51.
10. Lee CJ, Morasch MD. Treatment of vertebral disease: appropriate use of open and endovascular techniques. Semin Vasc Surg 2011;24:24–30.
11. Mehta S, Sharma P, Sridhar J. Flashes and Floaters. Urol Clin North Am 2015, in press.
12. Varma DD, Cugati S, Lee AW, et al. A review of central artery occlusion: clinical presentation and management. Eye (Lond) 2013;27:688–97.
13. Gonzalez-Gay MA, Pina T. Giant cell arteritis and polymyalgia rheumatic: an update. Curr Rheumatol Rep 2015;17:480.
14. Greven CM, Slusher MM, Weaver RG. Retinal arterial occlusions in young adults. Am J Ophthalmol 1995;120:776–83.
15. Newman-Casey PA, Stem M, Talwar N, et al. Risk factors associated with developing branch retinal vein occlusion among enrollees in a United States managed care plan. Ophthalmology 2014;121:1939–48.
16. Stern MS, Talwar N, Comer GM, et al. A longitudinal analysis of risk factors associated with central retinal vein occlusion. Ophthalmology 2013;120:362–70.
17. Risse F, Frank RD, Weinberger AW. Thrombophilia in patients with retinal vein occlusion: a retrospective analysis. Ophthalmologica 2014;232:46–52.
18. Khan Z, Almeida DR, Rahim K, et al. 10-Year Framingham risk in patients with retinal vein occlusion: a systematic review and meta-analysis. Can J Ophthalmol 2013;48:40–5.
19. Beck RW, Trobe JD. What we have learned from the Optic Neuritis Treatment Trial. Ophthalmology 1995;102:1504–8.

20. The Optic Neuritis Study Group. A randomized, controlled trial of corticosteroids in the treatment of acute optic neuritis. N Engl J Med 1992;326:581–8.

21. Boomer JA, Siatkowski RM. Optic neuritis in adults and children. Semin Ophthalmol 2003;18:174–80.

22. Kale N, Eggenberger E. Diagnosis and management of giant cell arteritis: a review. Curr Opin Ophthalmol 2010;21:417–22.

23. Hayreh SS. Ischemic optic neuropathies - where are we now? Graefes Arch Clin Exp Ophthalmol 2013;251:1873–84.

24. Atkins EJ, Bruce BB, Newman NJ, et al. Treatment of nonarteritic anterior ischemic optic neuropathy. Surv Ophthalmol 2010;55(1):47–63.

25. Hayreh SS. Role of nocturnal arterial hypotension in the development of ocular manifestations of systemic arterial hypertension. Curr Opin Ophthalmol 1999; 10:474–82.

26. Jeon SB, Koh Y, Choi HA, et al. Critical care for patients with massive ischemic stroke. J Stroke 2014;16:146–60.

27. Song S. Hyperacute management of ischemic stroke. Semin Neurol 2013;33: 427–35.

Corneal Abrasions and Corneal Foreign Bodies

Faheem Ahmed, MD[a], Robert James House, BA[b], Brad Hal Feldman, MD[c],*

KEYWORDS

- Corneal abrasion • Corneal foreign body • Management • Treatment

KEY POINTS

- Corneal abrasions and corneal foreign bodies have an incidence of approximately 3 and 2 per 1000 persons and represent a significant portion of ocular-related presentations to the emergency room.
- As many as one-quarter of all ocular injuries occur at the workplace and young males demonstrate the highest rates of occupational eye injuries.
- Both corneal abrasions and foreign bodies can have potentially sight-threatening consequences if not diagnosed and treated properly.
- A detailed history and thorough physical examination should be taken to rule out globe rupture or the presence of an intraocular foreign body.
- Referral to an ophthalmologist is recommended if the patient has signs and symptoms of a penetrating eye injury, corneal ulcer, recurrent erosion syndrome, a sight-threatening infection, or if the symptoms fail to improve after initial treatment.

INTRODUCTION

Corneal abrasions result from nonpenetrating defects to the epithelium of the cornea and account for a large percentage of ocular injuries seen by primary care physicians.[1,2] Patients can present with a foreign body sensation, severe pain, and sensitivity to light (photophobia), acute enough to require time away from work.[3] Although many cornea abrasions heal without treatment, serious complications can arise resulting in long-term damage and vision loss. Contact lens wear can cause mechanical injury to the cornea, as well as increased risk from virulent microbial pathogens.[4] Owing to the multitude of possible causes for corneal abrasions, it is important for primary care providers (PCPs) and emergency room (ER) physicians to understand the pathophysiology and etiology of a traumatic corneal injury. The role of the PCP

[a] Wills Eye Hospital, 840 Walnut Street, Philadelphia, PA 19107, USA; [b] San Juan Bautista School of Medicine, Caguas, PR 00727, USA; [c] Cornea Service, Wills Eye Hospital, 840 Walnut Street, Philadelphia, PA 19107, USA
* Corresponding author.
E-mail address: bradhfeldman@gmail.com

Prim Care Clin Office Pract 42 (2015) 363–375
http://dx.doi.org/10.1016/j.pop.2015.05.004
0095-4543/15/$ – see front matter © 2015 Elsevier Inc. All rights reserved.

or ER physician is to perform a detailed clinical history and comprehensive evaluation of the patient to initiate an appropriate intervention and determine if referral to an ophthalmologist is necessary.

EPIDEMIOLOGY
Frequency

Corneal abrasions and corneal foreign bodies are common and often preventable ocular injuries with an incidence of approximately 3 and 2 per 1000 persons, respectively, in the United States.[5] Eye-related diagnoses represent approximately 8% of total ER visits.[2] Of those eye-related occurrences, approximately 45% are corneal abrasions, followed by 31% from foreign bodies.[6] When researchers looked at patients presenting to an ophthalmic ER with a chief complaint of ocular foreign body sensation, 67.8% had a true corneal foreign body and 13.6% had a corneal abrasion.[7]

Work-Related Incidence and At-risk Populations

In a United Kingdom study of ER patients, 64% of patients diagnosed with a corneal abrasion had suffered direct minor trauma.[8] One of the most common causes of minor trauma in the pediatric and adult populations is chronic contact lens wear. According to Aslam and colleagues,[8] 12% of corneal abrasion cases were contact lens related. In a 6-month study conducted by Lee and colleagues,[9] 87% of patients who had contact lens–related trauma presented with epithelial staining, corneal abrasion, or epithelial defect (**Box 1**).

Some studies have reported that occupational eye injuries are responsible for at least one-quarter of all eye injuries, whereas other studies have demonstrated an even greater amount.[10] According to the 2008 Bureau of Labor Statistics[3] analysis of workplace injuries, occupational eye injuries account for 62% of facial injuries that lead to at least 1 day away from work. In this study, the sources of eye injury for almost one-half of all cases came from the category of scrap, waste, and debris.[3] The 3 primary manifestations of eye injuries from greatest to least were foreign bodies (34.2%), abrasions/scratches (14.9%), and chemical burns (10.4%).[3] The occurrence of ocular injuries in major industrial occupations were most common in construction and manufacturing jobs, which were responsible for 45% of all work-related eye injuries. The median number of days off from work with eye injuries was 2, with 44% of cases only involving a single day, and this compared favorably with the median of 8 days for all cases of work injury. These statistics demonstrate that, although corneal abrasions are relatively common, recovery time is much shorter than many other frequent work-related injuries.

Box 1
Risk factors for corneal abrasions

History of trauma (eg, direct blunt trauma, chemical burn, or radiation exposure)

Contact lens wear

Male gender

Age between 20 and 34 years old

Construction or manufacturing job

Lack of eye protection

Wong and colleagues[10] did a similar epidemiologic report of ocular injury over a 3-year span in several US car plants. Superficial foreign bodies and corneal abrasions were responsible for 87% of eye-related injuries. This study also demonstrated that only 25% of workers who had an ocular injury were wearing eye protection.[10] In this population, almost one-third of cases resulted in the worker needing at least 1 day off from resuming his or her normal workload.[10] This study suggests the preventability of corneal injury if workers are compliant with wearing protective eye gear in higher risk work environments. Other reports have demonstrated the effectiveness of eye protection in reducing eye injury in military combat.[11] In their retrospective study, Thomas and colleagues[11] reported that soldiers who wore military combat eye protection had a 9% reduction of ocular injury compared with soldiers not wearing protection at the time of injury. More importantly, the soldiers who were injured while wearing military combat eye protection had less severe injuries compared with their counterparts who wore no eye protection.[11]

Many studies regarding workplace eye injury rates report that young males have the highest rate of eye injury.[1,5] The 2008 Bureau of Labor Statistics data[3] found that as many as 81% of ocular injuries at work occur in men, compared with 63% of all workplace injuries. In the Bureau of Labor Statistics data, the highest incidence of occupational eye injury occurred in workers aged 25 to 34 years,[3] whereas Wong and colleagues[10] found the greatest incidence in workers aged 20 to 29 years old. The increased incidence of ocular injury for young males at the workplace might be based on the undertaking of more dangerous jobs, a disregard for safety measures, inexperience, or a combination of several factors.[10] Therefore, age and gender should be taken into consideration when examining patients with ocular emergencies[10] and when considering preventive counseling.

PRESENTATION

A corneal abrasion should be considered in the differential diagnosis whenever a patient presents with eye pain, red eye, tearing, decreased visual acuity, photophobia (sensitivity to light), foreign body sensation, or a history of trauma to the eye (**Box 2**).[2] Corneal injuries can result from blunt trauma—with fingernails[3] and contact lens wear being common causes[9]—foreign body entry, or chemical/radiation burns.[2,12]

A detailed history from the patient is very important in determining whether or not a corneal abrasion has occurred, and a proper diagnosis can help to direct the PCP and ER physician in their plan of treatment. Most patients will be able to recall a specific injury, although other patients will experience a summation of multiple injuries, as, for example, in aggressive eye rubbing or sleeping in contact lenses.[2] A corneal abrasion without a history of ocular injury can also be indicative of a more serious

Box 2
Presenting symptoms of corneal abrasions and foreign bodies
Eye pain
Watering/tearing
Decreased visual acuity
Photophobia (light sensitivity)
Red eye
Foreign body sensation

underlying issue, such as recurrent erosion syndrome,[2] staphylococcal marginal keratitis, infectious keratitis, or inflammatory keratitis. If the patient has a history of working with sharp metal or is unable to give a detailed history (as in the case of infants and toddlers), one must always consider the possibility of a penetrating eye injury.[2]

It is very important for the PCP and ER physician to be able to recognize and properly diagnose corneal abrasions because they can cause a great amount of pain, and can evolve into recurrent erosion syndrome, corneal ulcers, or sight-threatening infections.[1] Along with being able to provide basic ophthalmologic treatment, the PCP and ER physician should be able to judge when a patient should be referred to a specialist.[13] Although a PCP or ER physician can treat most corneal abrasions with ease, ophthalmic injuries can often be anxiety provoking for a non-ophthalmologist,[13] especially if they lack proper equipment or training to visualize the pathology under the slit lamp microscope.

EXAMINATION AND DIAGNOSIS

Despite their common prevalence, corneal abrasions and corneal foreign bodies may often be missed if the patient denies any recent trauma or does not seem to be in any significant discomfort. Therefore, a thorough clinical examination in conjunction with taking a detailed history is absolutely vital whenever there is suspected injury to the eye. In both the emergency and primary clinic settings, a stepwise systematic approach should be used to efficiently assess the visual function of the eyes.

An examination with a slit lamp and fluorescein dye is ideal to properly document the depth and size of suspected abrasions.[8] A slit lamp, however, may not be accessible to the PCP or ER physician. Therefore, the following materials should be readily available to perform a comprehensive eye examination: a Snellen visual acuity chart, penlight, a direct ophthalmoscope or Wood's lamp, topical anesthetic drops, and fluorescein strips. The patient's monocular visual acuity should be documented for each eye with a handheld Snellen visual acuity chart, which readily can be printed off the Internet or displayed on a mobile device. If a significant change from baseline vision is detected in the affected eye (eg, patient is now hand motion or light perception in a previously normal eye), then immediate ophthalmology referral is warranted. Otherwise, a transient decrease in visual acuity is to be expected, especially if the corneal abrasion is located in the central visual axis. The patient's extraocular motility should also be checked. If there is a deficit, there may be entrapment of the muscle or a nerve palsy that may require emergent imaging to rule out an orbital fracture.

After documenting the visual acuity, a penlight can be used to scan the ocular adnexa of the affected eye, including the lids, conjunctiva, and orbit for any signs of inflammation or trauma. The upper eyelids should be everted to check for the presence of a foreign body (**Fig. 1**).[14] If the history includes high-velocity impact as the mechanism of injury to the eye, there may be extrusion of ocular contents or the pupil may be dilated, nonreactive or irregular. Emergent ophthalmology referral is necessary in these cases to rule out an open globe rupture. In a majority of corneal abrasions, however, the pupil is round and reactive, and the light reflex is unaffected.

Owing to the dense innervation of the cornea, patients with abrasions are typically in moderate to great discomfort. A single drop of topical ophthalmic anesthetic such as proparacaine can be applied to the corneal surface to temporarily alleviate pain in order to facilitate proper examination, but should not be given repeatedly for pain management as this will hinder the healing response.[14] The bulbar conjunctiva is often injected and there will be reflex tearing owing to irritation. Ciliary spasm

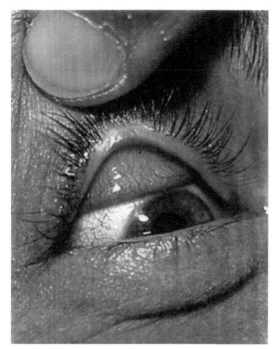

Fig. 1. Foreign body present on eversion of right upper lid. (*Courtesy of* American Academy of Ophthalmology © 2014; with permission.)

induced meiosis of the pupil and hyperemia of the ciliary vessels surrounding the cornea (limbal flush) may indicate additional traumatic iritis.[2] If there is a hazy appearance to the cornea and the light reflex is dull, there may be corneal edema owing to blunt trauma or excessive rubbing. Discovery of a foreign body lodged in the cornea, regardless of material or depth, requires an ophthalmologist for removal at a slit lamp (**Fig. 2**). Next, the penlight should be used to examine grossly the depth

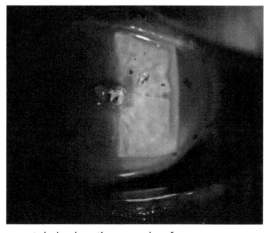

Fig. 2. Metallic fragments lodged on the corneal surface.

and clarity of the anterior chamber. Evidence of frank blood in the anterior chamber (hyphema) or purulent fluid (hypopyon) also requires immediate ophthalmologic referral.[2]

Corneal abrasions are often very subtle and can be missed with unaided visual inspection using a penlight (**Fig. 3**). Therefore, fluorescein dye is a necessary tool to diagnose any occult corneal epithelial defect.[12] Fluorescein is available as an eye drop mixed with a topical anesthetic or as fluorescein paper strips. These strips are moistened with a drop of topical anesthetic, artificial tear solution, or saline solution and then gently touched to the inferior conjunctival sac. The dye spreads over the cornea as the patient blinks. Fluorescein does not penetrate intact conjunctival or corneal epithelium, but readily stains exposed corneal stroma or basement membrane. Using the cobalt blue filter on a direct ophthalmoscope or a Wood's lamp, the cornea will be illuminated and any epithelial defect will fluoresce a bright green color (**Fig. 4**).

The differential diagnosis for a corneal epithelial defect includes the following (**Box 3**): trauma, herpes simplex virus, neurotrophia, exposure keratopathy, recurrent erosion, postoperative complication, chemical exposure, ultraviolet (UV) exposure, dry eye, limbal stem cell deficiency, trichiasis, and keratoconjunctivitis. Traumatic corneal abrasions will appear as linear or geographic lesions.[2] Herpes simplex virus keratitis classically appears as a dendritic pattern with terminal bulbs, but can be geographic as well and mimic a large corneal abrasion. A neurotrophic erosion typically appears as a geographic epithelial defect with rolled edges on the central or inferior cornea and should be suspected in patients with damage to the corneal nerves. This includes patients with a history of diabetic neuropathy, after infection with varicella zoster virus or herpes simplex virus, chronic contact lens wear, or abuse of topical anesthetics.

Exposure keratopathy should be suspected in patients with incomplete lid closure, termed lagophthalmos, which is commonly seen in Bell's palsy, or infrequent blink, which is commonly associated with Parkinson's disease. Recurrent corneal erosions often appear in the central cornea with loose epithelium that shifts upon blinking. These patients may relate a history of recurrent pain upon awakening. Chemical and UV keratitis occur after accidental exposure, and although the pain from chemical injury is immediate, UV-related symptoms typically begin hours after exposure. Limbal

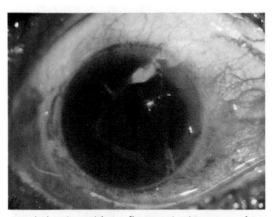

Fig. 3. Traumatic corneal abrasion without fluorescein. (*Courtesy of* American Academy of Ophthalmology © 2014; with permission.)

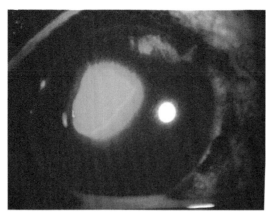

Fig. 4. Corneal abrasion with fluorescein stain viewed under cobalt blue light. (*Courtesy of* American Academy of Ophthalmology © 2014; with permission.)

stem cell deficiency is a chronic condition that leads to poor wound healing and spontaneous corneal abrasions. Corneal abrasions and chronic scarring plus the evidence of misdirected eyelashes toward the globe are highly suggestive of trichiasis, which is endemic in many parts of the developing world. Establishing the etiology of the corneal defect helps to guide the management of symptoms and appropriate referrals, and ensures proper treatment for the patient.

TREATMENT

The goals of treatment with corneal abrasions are to prevent bacterial superinfection, speed healing, and to provide symptomatic relief to patients (**Fig. 5**). Although the cornea is a resilient tissue that often heals without complication, any epithelial defect puts the cornea at risk from pathogenic infection. Therefore, the mainstay of treatment in all corneal abrasions is antibiotic prophylaxis with either lubricating ointments, topical drops, or a combination of both therapies. If the mechanism of injury to the cornea involves contact lens wear, fingernails, or vegetable/organic plant matter,

---

Box 3
Differential diagnosis of corneal abrasions

Trauma (work related, postoperative, contact lens wear)

Infectious keratitis (bacterial, fungal, herpetic)

Neutrotrophia

Exposure keratopathy

Limbal stem cell deficiency

Environmental (chemical, ultraviolet light)

Recurrent erosion syndrome

Dry eye syndrome

Trichiasis

Keratoconjunctivitis

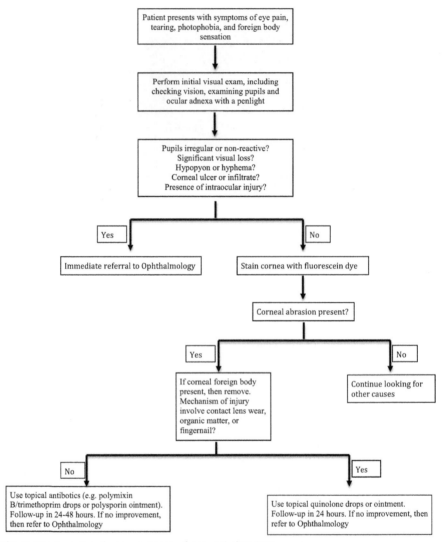

Fig. 5. Treatment and management of corneal abrasions.

antibiotic prophylaxis should be provided with topical fluoroquinolone drops (eg, ofloxacin or moxifloxacin) at least 4 times a day, and typically a fluoroquinolone ointment (eg, ciprofloxacin) at night time to provide coverage against gram-negative organisms.

Patients who are chronic contact lens wearers often are colonized with *Pseudomonas aeruginosa*, which is notorious for causing rapid corneal perforation and subsequent permanent vision loss.[2] Fluoroquinolones are advantageous because of their broad-spectrum coverage and low toxicity. If the mechanism of injury does not involve contact lens wear or organic plant matter, treatment options include administration of antibiotic ointments (eg, erythromycin, bacitracin, or polysporin every 2 or 4 hours), or with antibiotic drops (eg, polymyxin B and trimethoprim or fluoroquinolone 4 times a day).

For patients complaining of significant pain and discomfort, options for pain relief include oral analgesics such as acetaminophen or nonsteroidal antiinflammatory drugs, topical cycloplegics, and rarely opioid analgesics in severe cases. Patients with photophobia and ciliary spasm secondary to traumatic iritis tend to have rapid relief of symptoms with cycloplegics, such as cyclopentolate 1%, 2 to 3 times a day. Topical nonsteroidal antiinflammatory drugs should not be offered to patients with corneal abrasions owing to the risk of corneal toxicity.[15] Although topical anesthesia can be used to aid with physician examination, extended use of topical anesthetics is absolutely contraindicated with any corneal injury. Repeated administration of topical anesthetics has been shown to delay corneal wound healing, mask worsening symptoms such as development of a corneal ulcer, and can also be toxic to corneal epithelium.[16] Similarly, topical steroids should be avoided in initial management.

In years past, physicians have often turned to treating traumatic corneal abrasions with pressure patching or a bandage contact lens in the affected eye. Recent studies, however, have shown that there is no advantage in the use of pressure patches or bandage contact lenses over antibiotic prophylaxis alone in terms of reducing the abrasion area and reducing pain.[17] Furthermore, pressure patching may do more patient harm by removing binocular vision and, in some cases, increasing patient pain and discomfort.[18] Similarly, the use of bandage contact lenses should be avoided owing to the potential incubation of pathogenic organisms and promoting subsequent infectious keratitis.

COMPLICATIONS

Although a majority of corneal abrasions heal within 2 to 3 days without issue, some can potentially develop long-term, sight-threatening complications if treated improperly. Corneal foreign bodies, if not removed promptly by an ophthalmologist, can cause repeated damage to the cornea and lead to chronic scarring and a subsequent permanent decrease in visual function. Metallic foreign bodies, for example, if not completely removed from the corneal tissue, can leave behind rust rings that delay wound healing. Other complications of corneal abrasion include corneal ulcer, bacterial keratitis, recurrent erosion, and traumatic iritis.

A corneal ulcer is defined as a defect of the epithelium with involvement or loss of the underlying stroma (**Fig. 6**). The associated inflammation can be either sterile or secondary to infectious pathogens. Sterile infiltrates are much more common and typically benign self-limited conditions, representing a low-grade immune response to bacterial exotoxins (eg, *Staphylococcus aureus*). Infectious microbial ulcers, on the other hand, are much more rare, but can lead to sight-threatening keratitis. Patients who use extended wear contact lens can increase their risk of microbial keratitis by 15 times, and patients who wear their daily wear contact lens occasionally at night increase their risk of developing microbial keratitis by 9 times.[9] Signs of an infectious corneal ulcer include a visible white or discolored infiltrate in the anterior cornea or pus in the anterior chamber (hypopyon).

Another long-term complication of corneal abrasion is recurrent erosions. Erosions typically are first felt upon awakening, may occur days to years after the initial abrasion heals, and seem to be similar to a corneal abrasion when stained with fluorescein. These recurrent cases should be referred to an ophthalmologist to seek further treatment (**Box 4**).

In the hospital environment, perioperative corneal abrasions can occur, with the most notable risk factors being advanced patient age, use of general anesthesia, patient positioning, and use of oxygen in the transport and recovery process.[19] ER

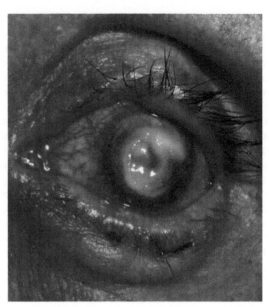

Fig. 6. Infectious central corneal ulcer. Immediate referral to ophthalmology is necessary. (*Courtesy of* American Academy of Ophthalmology © 2014; with permission.)

and hospital-based personnel should be aware that postoperative patients complaining of blurry vision, tearing, redness, photophobia, and foreign body sensation could be presenting with the clinical symptoms of corneal abrasion.[19] Neonatal patients using mask ventilation are also a high-risk population, and eye discharge can be a sign of infection and possible corneal abrasion.[20]

PREVENTION

Prevention is the most logical and cost-effective method for treating corneal abrasions and the potential long-term complications that can develop. Protective eyewear should be used for all persons who work with machinery, metal, wood, or chemicals. People who perform yard work (eg, mowing the lawn, trimming branches), housework (eg, pounding with a hammer, using hazardous cleaning

---

Box 4
Reasons for immediate referral to an ophthalmologist

- Signs or symptoms of penetrating eye injury or globe rupture
  - Presentation of a dilated, nonreactive, or irregular pupil
  - Blood (hyphema) or purulent fluid (hypopyon) in the anterior chamber
- Discovery of a foreign body in the cornea
- Recurrent episodes of corneal abrasion or ulcer
- Evidence of other secondary complications, such as bacterial keratitis or traumatic iritis
- Failure to improve 24 to 48 hours after initial treatment

supplies), as well as people who participate in certain contact sports, paintballing, playing with fireworks, and other potentially high-risk activity should also wear eye protection. The appropriate type of protective eyewear depends on the specific circumstances, but all should provide proper shielding, good visibility, and a comfortable fit.

Polycarbonate glasses or goggles, plastic safety glasses, face shields, and welding helmets are examples of eyewear that can offer a protective barrier and help to prevent corneal abrasions and foreign bodies getting embedded in the eye. Specifically, welders should use a helmet with a lens that blocks UV light to avoid UV keratitis. Monocular patients are especially vulnerable to blinding injuries, and should pay special attention to protecting their eyes by using polycarbonate glasses in any activity where a sharp or blunt object could possibly injure the eye. In these cases, protective eyewear can ensure some degree of safety while also allowing patients to participate in their normal day-to-day activities.

Ensuring that contact lenses fit well on the cornea, and encouraging patient compliance with wearing their contact lenses as directed, can prevent corneal abrasions from contact lens-related complications. Proper care and maintenance of contact lenses and their accessories are essential to preventing corneal damage, because the greatest risk factor for developing microbial keratitis is contact lens wear, particularly in extended wear contacts with hydrogel lenses.[4] Many factors contribute to the increased risk of microbial keratitis, with the primary associations being overnight contact lens wear and poor lens hygiene.[9] Contact lens solution and lens cases are also sources of potentially pathogenic microbes, with the possibility of bacterial colonization leading to antimicrobial resistant biofilm in contact lens cases.[4] An emphasis should be placed on reducing lens contamination by using effective disinfecting solution, as well as antimicrobial contact lenses and cases.[4] It is important to avoid swimming with contact lenses, because this increases the frequency of bacterial infections, primarily from *Staphylococcus epidermidis* and other organisms found in chlorinated pools or contaminated water.[4] Patients who use contact lenses can also avoid both mechanical and infectious trauma by not using contacts beyond the length of their intended use (eg, wearing monthly contacts for >1 month). All of these recommendations also apply to the use of cosmetic contact lenses, which should be fitted properly by an eye care professional and cared for on a daily basis.

SUMMARY

Corneal abrasions and corneal foreign bodies have an incidence of approximately 3 and 2 per 1000 persons, respectively, in the United States, and represent a significant portion of ocular-related presentations to the ER. As many as one-quarter of all ocular injuries, occur at the workplace and young males demonstrate the highest rates of occupational eye injuries. Patients with contact lenses also have an increased risk of developing a corneal abrasion, especially if the contact lenses do not fit properly and are not used as directed. Both corneal abrasions and foreign bodies can have potentially sight-threatening consequences if not diagnosed and treated properly.

Although many corneal abrasions heal in 2 to 3 days without issue, possible secondary complications include corneal ulcer, recurrent erosions, and traumatic iritis. If not properly removed, long-term risks of a corneal foreign body include repeated mechanical damage to the cornea, chronic scarring, the presence of rust rings that can delay healing, and subsequent vision loss. Patients who are diagnosed with a corneal abrasion or foreign body should be treated with prophylactic antibiotics, such as lubricating ointment, topical drops, or a combination of both therapies, as well as oral analgesics if they are experiencing significant pain and discomfort. A detailed patient history should always be performed along with a thorough physical examination to rule out the possibility of a globe rupture or the presence of an intraocular foreign body. If the history includes a high-velocity traumatic injury with a pupil that is dilated, nonreactive, or irregular, then emergent ophthalmology referral is necessary. Referral to an ophthalmologist is recommended in difficult cases or if the patient has signs and symptoms of a penetrating eye injury, corneal ulcer, recurrent erosion syndrome, a sight-threatening infection, or if the symptoms fail to improve after initial treatment.

REFERENCES

1. Lin YB, Gardiner MF. Fingernail-induced corneal abrasions: case series from an ophthalmology emergency department. Cornea 2014;33(7):691–5.
2. Wipperman JL, Dorsch JN. Evaluation and management of corneal abrasions. Am Fam Physician 2013;87(2):114–20.
3. Harris PM. Bureau of Labor Statistics. Workplace injuries involving the eyes, 2008. 2011. Available at: http://www.bls.gov/opub/mlr/cwc/workplace-injuries-involving-the-eyes-2008.pdf. Accessed September 6, 2014.
4. Szczotka-Flynn LB, Pearlman E, Ghannoum M. Microbial contamination of contact lenses, lens care solutions, and their accessories: a literature review. Eye Contact Lens 2010;36(2):116–29.
5. McGwin G Jr, Xie A, Owsley C. Rate of eye injury in the United States. Arch Ophthalmol 2005;123(7):970–6.
6. McGwin G, Owsley C. Incidence of emergency department-treated eye injury in the United States. Arch Ophthalmol 2005;123:662–6.
7. Jayamanne DG. Do patients presenting to accident and emergency departments with the sensation of a foreign body in the eye (gritty eye) have significant ocular disease? J Accid Emerg Med 1995;12:286–7.
8. Aslam SA, Sheth HG, Vaughan AJ. Emergency management of corneal injuries. Injury 2007;38:594–7.
9. Lee SY, Kim YH, Johnson D, et al. Contact lens complications in an urgent-care population: the University of California, Los Angeles, contact lens study. Eye Contact Lens 2012;38(1):49–52.
10. Wong TY, Lincoln A, Tielsch JM, et al. The epidemiology of ocular injury in a major US automobile corporation. Eye (Lond) 1998;12:870–4.
11. Thomas R, McManus JG, Johnson A, et al. Ocular injury reduction from ocular protection use in current combat operations. J Trauma 2009;66(4 Suppl):S99–103.
12. Khaw PT, Shah P, Elkington AR. ABC of eyes. Injury to the eye. BMJ 2004;328: 36–8.
13. Thyagarajan SK, Sharma V, Austin S, et al. An audit of corneal abrasion management following the introduction of local guidelines in an accident and emergency department. Emerg Med J 2006;23:526–9.
14. Shahid SM, Harrison N. Corneal abrasion: assessment and management. InnovAiT 2013;6(9):551–4.
15. Kim SJ, Flach AJ, Jampol LM. Nonsteroidal anti-inflammatory drugs in ophthalmology. Surv Ophthalmol 2010;55(2):108–33.
16. Duffin RM, Olson RJ. Tetracaine toxicity. Ann Ophthalmol 1984;16(9):836–8.
17. Menghini M, Knecht PB, Kaufmann C, et al. Treatment of traumatic corneal abrasions: a three-arm, prospective, randomized study. Ophthalmic Res 2013; 50:13–8.

18. Flynn CA, D'Amico F, Smith G. Should we patch corneal abrasions? A meta-analysis. J Fam Pract 1998;47(4):264–70.
19. Segal KL, Fleischut PM, Kim C, et al. Evaluation and treatment of perioperative corneal abrasions. J Ophthalmol 2014;2014:1–5.
20. Wilson SA, Last A. Management of corneal abrasions. Am Fam Physician 2004; 70(1):123–8.

Age-Related Macular Degeneration

Sonia Mehta, MD

KEYWORDS

- Age-related macular degeneration
- Nonexudative age-related macular degeneration • Dry AMD
- Exudative age-related macular degeneration • Wet AMD
- Neovascular age-related macular degeneration

KEY POINTS

- Age-related macular degeneration (AMD) is the leading cause of vision loss in the elderly.
- AMD causes loss of central vision over time. It does not cause complete blindness because peripheral vision is generally unaffected in this disease.
- Dry AMD is characterized by the presence of age-related deposits called drusen and atrophy.
- In addition to drusen and atrophy, wet AMD is characterized by the presence of edema and hemorrhage within or below the retina or retinal pigment epithelium.
- Early detection and treatment of AMD is crucial to improving likelihood for patients in retaining good and functional vision.

INTRODUCTION
Disease Description

Age-related macular degeneration (AMD) is an acquired degeneration of the retina that can cause central vision problems through nonneovascular (drusen and atrophy) and neovascular derangement (choroidal neovascular membranes).

Definition

AMD is a clinical diagnosis based on characteristic findings on dilated retinal examination in patients ages 50 years and older. These findings are localized to the center of the retina (macula) and include extensive small drusen, intermediate or large drusen, geographic atrophy, choroidal neovascularization, or disciform scar formation.

Vitreoretinal Diseases & Surgery Service, Wills Eye Hospital, Department of Ophthalmology, Thomas Jefferson University Hospital, 840 Walnut Street, Suite 1020, Philadelphia, PA 19107, USA
E-mail address: soniamehtamd@gmail.com

Prim Care Clin Office Pract 42 (2015) 377–391
http://dx.doi.org/10.1016/j.pop.2015.05.009   primarycare.theclinics.com
0095-4543/15/$ – see front matter © 2015 Elsevier Inc. All rights reserved.

Prevalence and Incidence

The prevalence of AMD is 9.2% in persons 50 years and older in the United States.[1] The prevalence of AMD differs among different ethnic groups (**Table 1**).[1,2] In comparison, the prevalence of diabetic retinopathy in persons 40 years and older in the United States is 3.4%.[3] AMD is more prevalent in individuals older than 60 years of age compared with persons in their fifth or sixth decades of life.[2] Although dry AMD accounts for 85% to 90% of AMD, wet AMD causes 90% of severe vision loss from AMD.[4]

Risk factors for AMD are described in **Table 2**. Patients interested in the prevention of AMD should be advised to not start or quit smoking and to eat a diet rich in antioxidants such as β-carotene, vitamin C, vitamin E, and zinc.[5,6] In addition, patients can wear appropriate sunglasses outdoors to block ultraviolet and blue light that can cause eye damage.[7]

Symptom Criteria

Patients with AMD may complain of the following symptoms:

- Decreased vision;
- Blurry vision;
- Metamorphopsia (distortion of central vision, straight lines appearing wavy); and
- Central scotomas (areas of lost vision).

Patients complaining of vision loss should be referred to ophthalmology. Patients with acute vision loss should be sent for urgent ophthalmologic evaluation.

CLINICAL FINDINGS
Physical Examination

Early in the disease, visual acuity may be normal and vision may be unaffected. In dry AMD, also known as nonexudative AMD, dilated fundus examination reveals macular

Table 1 Prevalence of age-related macular degeneration in the US population	
Variable	**%**
General US population	9.2
Ethnicity	
Non-Hispanic white	9.3
Black	7.4
Hispanic	7.1
Age (y)	
50–54	0.4
55–59	0.4
60–64	0.6
65–69	0.9
70–74	1.6
75–79	3.1
>80	11.7

Data from Klein R, Rowland ML, Harris MI. Racial/ethnic differences in age-related maculopathy. Third National Health and Nutrition Examination Survey. Ophthalmology 1995;102:371–81; and 2010 U.S. age-specific prevalence rates for AMD by age, and race/ethnicity. Available at: https://nei.nih.gov/eyedata/amd. Accessed January 3, 2015.

Table 2
Risk factors for age-related macular degeneration (AMD)

Factor	Impact
Age	The prevalence of AMD increases with age.[2]
Ethnicity	The prevalence of AMD is greater in non-Hispanic whites than in blacks or Hispanic populations.[1,2]
Smoking	The risk of developing AMD is 2 times more likely in smokers than nonsmokers. In addition, in patients with AMD, wet AMD is 3 times more likely in smokers compared with nonsmokers.[5]
Genetics	The role of genetics in AMD is under study and is not yet defined. Genetic factors are more directly related to early onset macular degenerations in younger individuals; this condition is separate from AMD.
Diet	High dietary intakes of antioxidants such as β-carotene, vitamin C, vitamin E, and zinc have been associated with a decreased risk of AMD in older individuals.[6]
Sun exposure	Patients with increased sun exposure are at increased risk of developing AMD.[7]

Data from Refs.[1,2,5–7]

drusen, which are yellowish age-related deposits between Bruch's membrane and the retinal pigment epithelium (**Fig. 1**). Drusen are thought to be secondary to retinal pigment epithelial dysfunction.[8,9]

In dry AMD, as the disease progresses, retinal examination is characterized by geographic atrophy, which is a thinning of the retinal pigment epithelium and overlying retina (**Fig. 2**). Wet AMD, also known as neovascular or exudative AMD, is characterized by choroidal neovascularization in which patients can have subretinal fluid or intraretinal fluid (**Fig. 3**). Patients can also have hemorrhage below the retina or the retinal pigment epithelium. This can progress to fibrosis underneath the retina that, when extensive, is known as disciform scarring (**Fig. 4**).

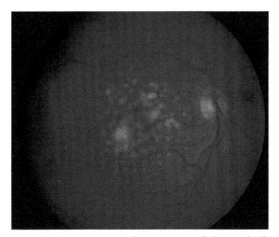

Fig. 1. Fundus photograph demonstrating the presence of drusen (yellow deposits) in dry age-related macular degeneration.

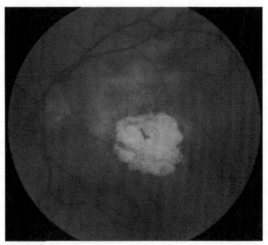

Fig. 2. Fundus photograph demonstrating the presence of geographic atrophy in advanced dry age-related macular degeneration.

Rating Scales

The most commonly used classification system for AMD is based on the Age-Related Eye Disease Study (AREDS).[10]

- No AMD (AREDS category 1): None or few small drusen (<63 microns).
- Early AMD (AREDS category 2): Multiple small drusen, few intermediate drusen (63–124 microns), or retinal pigment epithelium abnormalities.
- Intermediate AMD (AREDS category 3): Extensive intermediate drusen, 1 large druse (>125 microns), or geographic atrophy not involving the center of the fovea.

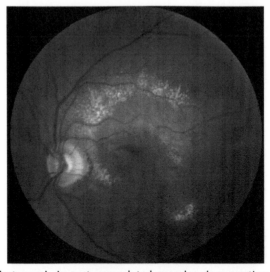

Fig. 3. Fundus photograph in wet age-related macular degeneration showing edema, subretinal fluid, and subretinal hemorrhage in the macula.

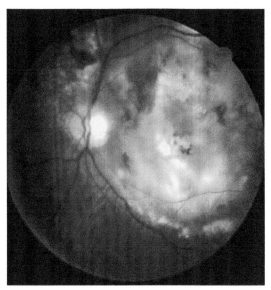

Fig. 4. Fundus photograph demonstrating scar tissue in the macula advanced wet age-related macular degeneration.

- Advanced AMD (AREDS category 4): Geographic atrophy involving the center of the fovea or any of the features associated with neovascular AMD, such as choroidal neovascularization or disciform scarring.

Diagnostic Modalities

Optical coherence tomography is a very useful modality in the diagnosis and management of AMD. This noninvasive imaging test performed in ophthalmology clinics displays detailed cross-sectional images of the retina. This imaging modality helps to identify areas of fluid or hemorrhage below or within the retina and also the retinal pigment epithelium (**Fig. 5**). In addition, the test reveals drusen and areas of retinal and retinal pigment epithelial thinning as seen in dry AMD (**Fig. 6**).

Fundus autofluorescence is a diagnostic imaging test used to detect the presence of fluorophores in the retina.[11] Fluorophores are chemical compounds that reemit light upon being exposed to light at a specific wavelength. In this noninvasive imaging modality, the natural fluorophores present in the fundus emit fluorescence when excited by light and the emitted fluorescence is captured and processed into images. Fundus autofluorescence also detects lipofuscin, a metabolic waste product found in many

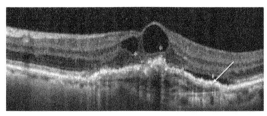

Fig. 5. Optical coherence tomography in wet age-related macular degeneration demonstrating the presence of fluid below (*arrow*) and in (*asterisks*) the retina.

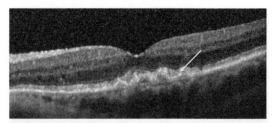

Fig. 6. Optical coherence tomography in dry age-related macular degeneration demonstrating the presence of drusen (*arrow*) at the level of the retinal pigment epithelium.

organs, including the eye, that is increased in patients with AMD. Fundus autofluorescence can also be used as a marker for the health of the retinal pigment epithelium.[11] Fundus autofluorescence is very useful in demonstrating the extent of geographic atrophy in dry AMD and following its progression over time (**Fig. 7**).

Fluorescein angiography is helpful in determining whether a patient has the exudative form of the disease. In this test, fluorescein dye is injected via the antecubital vein. A camera takes fundus photographs as the dye circulates through the retinal and choroidal vasculature. If an abnormal neovascular membrane is present, the dye circulates throughout the membrane with leakage later in the angiogram (**Fig. 8**).

Comorbidities

Additional age-related eye diseases such as cataract can be seen in patients with AMD.[12] The Beaver Dam Eye Study reported the relative risk of developing early AMD over 10 years associated with cataract at baseline was 1.3.[12] Even in patients with advanced AMD, cataract extraction may provide visual benefit by improving contrast sensitivity, brightness, and color.[13,14]

One study comparing wet AMD patients with age-, gender-, and race-matched controls found that individuals with wet AMD were significantly more likely to have comorbidities such as hypertension, hypercholesterolemia, emphysema, chronic obstructive

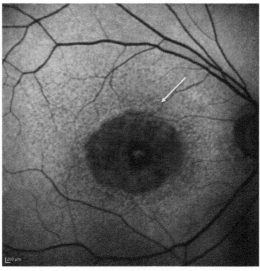

Fig. 7. Fundus autofluorescence in dry age-related macular degeneration demonstrating decreased autofluorescence in the macula from the presence of geographic atrophy (*arrow*).

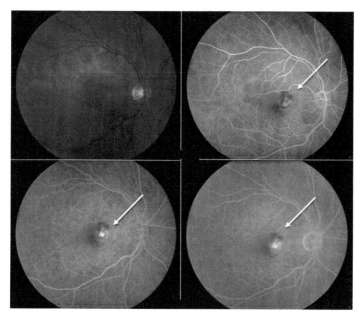

Fig. 8. Fluorescein angiogram in wet age-related macular degeneration demonstrating leakage from a choroidal neovascular membrane (*arrows*).

pulmonary disease, atherosclerosis, arthritis, and coronary heart disease. In addition, patients with wet AMD were found to more likely have cataract, glaucoma, and myopia compared with age-matched controls.[15]

Management Goals

The main principle in the management of dry AMD is to slow the progression of vision loss and to optimize the vision the patient has with use of visual aids. In wet AMD, the latest treatments have not only allowed ophthalmologists to slow down the progression of vision loss, but also to gain vision and improve visual acuity. Early diagnosis and treatment are key in optimizing the result for vision.[16]

Referral Strategies

The US Preventative Services Task Force and the American Academy of Family Physicians recommend visual acuity testing with the Snellen eye chart in elderly patients.[17,18] However, the US Preventative Services Task Force maintains that there is insufficient evidence to recommend a specific frequency of screening, screening questions, or screening ophthalmoscopy.

The American Academy of Ophthalmology recommends comprehensive eye examinations including a dilated fundus examination every year in patients greater than 55 years old in patients who do not have eye conditions requiring intervention.[19] Any patients complaining of vision loss should be referred to ophthalmology. Patients with acute vision loss should be sent for urgent evaluation.

PHARMACOLOGIC STRATEGIES
Age-Related Early Disease Study Vitamin Supplements

If an individual has intermediate or advanced AMD in one eye then use of AREDS vitamin supplements can slow the progression of the disease.[10] AREDS demonstrated that use of AREDS vitamins in patients with intermediate or unilateral advanced AMD slowed the progression of intermediate AMD to advanced AMD by 25% and decreased risk of vision loss by 19%. The AREDS dietary supplement consists of a daily dose of 500 mg vitamin C, 400 IU of vitamin E, 15 mg β-carotene, 80 mg of zinc oxide, and 2 mg cupric oxide. Because 80 mg of zinc oxide intake can result in copper deficiency, 2 mg of cupric oxide was added to the AREDS formula to prevent anemia from copper deficiency. A follow-up study showed that use of AREDS2 vitamin supplements in patients with intermediate or advanced AMD slowed the progression of intermediate to advanced AMD by 18% more than when compared with the original AREDS formula.[20] The AREDS2 dietary supplement consists of 500 mg vitamin C, 400 IU of vitamin E, 10 mg lutein, 2 mg zeaxanthin, 80 mg of zinc oxide, and 2 mg of cupric oxide for prevention of copper deficiency anemia.

Patients should check with their physicians before starting the AREDS or AREDS2 dietary supplements to make sure there is no contraindication to using this formula of antioxidants. Patients who are smokers should be informed that higher doses of β-carotene can result in an increased risk of developing lung cancer.[21] One study observed an 18% greater incidence of lung cancer among male smokers who received β-carotene compared with male smokers who did not receive β-carotene.[21] Therefore, it is common practice to advise smokers or previous smokers who have AMD to use the AREDS2 formula or AREDS vitamin supplements without β-carotene.

Anti-Vascular Endothelial Growth Factor

In patients with wet AMD, anti-vascular endothelial growth factor (VEGF) medication given as an intravitreal injection has revolutionized the treatment of wet AMD. VEGF contributes to angiogenesis by binding to its receptor on endothelial cells leading to endothelial cell proliferation and new blood vessel growth. Anti-VEGF is an antibody to the VEGF molecule. Anti-VEGF binds to soluble VEGF and inhibits the binding of VEGF to its receptor thereby inhibiting angiogenesis. This results in decreased activity of the choroidal neovascular membrane, which results in decreased intraretinal fluid, subretinal fluid, and subretinal hemorrhage in patients with wet AMD (**Fig. 9**).

Bevacizumab (Avastin, Genentech, San Francisco, CA), ranibizumab (Lucentis, Genentech), and aflibercept (Eylea, Regeneron Pharmaceuticals Inc, Tarrytown, NY) are the 3 anti-VEGF medications used in the treatment of wet AMD. These medications are given as an intravitreal injection through the conjunctiva, sclera, and into the vitreous of the eye. The intravitreal injection is typically given every 4 weeks. The typical amount given is 0.05 mL and dose varies based on medication (1.25 mg bevacizumab, 0.5 mg ranibizumab, or 2 mg aflibercept). Both ranibizumab and aflibercept are approved by the US Food and Drug Administration for the treatment of wet AMD. While Bevacizumab is not approved by the US Food and Drug Administration for ocular use; however, it is used commonly to treat wet AMD off label.

Several large clinical trials have been performed demonstrating the efficacy of anti-VEGF medications in the treatment of AMD.[22–27] The Minimally Classic/Occult Trial of the Anti-VEGF antibody Ranibizumab in the treatment of Neovascular Age-Related Macular Degeneration (MARINA) trial compared sham injection with ranibizumab injections in the treatment of wet AMD.[23] Patients in the sham injection showed vision loss of 14.9 letters from baseline over 2 years, whereas patients in the treated group gained 6.6 letters in vision on average over 2 years. The Comparison of Age-Related Macular Degeneration Treatments Trials (CATT) and Inhibit VEGF in the Age-Related Choroidal Neovascularization trial (IVAN) were large clinical trials comparing ranibizumab and bevacizumab in the treatment of wet AMD.[24,25] Both studies showed that patients undergoing treatment with ranibizumab and bevacizumab gained 8.8 and

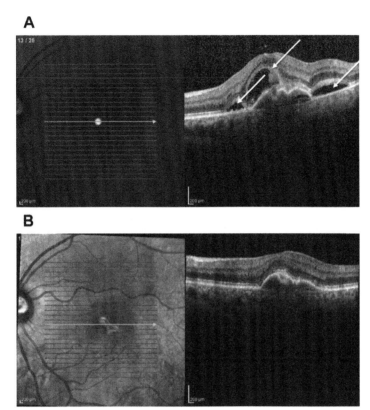

Fig. 9. (*A*) Optical coherence tomography of a patient with wet age-related macular degeneration before treatment. Note the presence of fluid below the retina (*arrows*). (*B*) Optical coherence tomography of the same patient following intravitreal Lucentis injections. Note that the fluid below the retina has resolved.

7.8 letters, respectively, in vision on average over 2 years. The CATT and IVAN trials showed no difference in the treatment effect between these 2 drugs in AMD. The VEGF Trap Investigation of Efficacy and Safety in wet AMD (VIEW) studies compared aflibercept and ranibizumab in the treatment of wet AMD.[26,27] VIEW 1 and VIEW 2 demonstrated that patients undergoing treatment with aflibercept gained 7.6 letters of vision on average over 2 years. VIEW 1 and VIEW 2 demonstrated that aflibercept was clinically equivalent to ranibizumab in the treatment of wet AMD.

NONPHARMACOLOGIC STRATEGIES
Laser Photocoagulation

Before anti-VEGF therapy, laser photocoagulation of the choroidal neovascular membranes had been performed to prevent severe vision loss in patients with wet AMD. However, laser photocoagulation is associated with high recurrence rates and can induce vision loss, especially when used to treat subfoveal choroidal neovascular membranes.[28,29] Furthermore, laser treatment fails to improve vision in patients with wet AMD. Therefore, in the era where anti-VEGF treatment is widely available, laser photocoagulation currently has limited use in the treatment of wet AMD.

Photodynamic Therapy

Before anti-VEGF, photodynamic therapy (PDT) was also a popular treatment for wet AMD. In this treatment, a photosensitive dye, verteporfin (Visudyne) is injected into the bloodstream via a peripheral vein. The verteporfin pools in neovascular membranes. When a laser treatment is applied to the neovascular membrane, the verteporfin is excited. The activated dye then forms reactive free radicals that damage the neovascular membrane, reducing the stimulus for leakage and bleeding below the retina. Because the normal retinal vasculature retains little dye, the abnormal neovascular membrane is selectively treated and sustains damage. After PDT, patients have to avoid exposure to the sun and sources of bright light. Similar to laser photocoagulation, although this treatment helps to prevent vision loss in wet AMD, PDT is associated with a high recurrent rate and failure to improve vision in patients with wet AMD.[30] Since the development of anti-VEGF, PDT is used less commonly in the treatment of wet AMD. However, this treatment is still used in patients with wet AMD with incomplete response to anti-VEGF therapy or to reduce treatment burden in patients unable to come in for monthly or frequent intravitreal anti-VEGF injections.

Low Vision Aids

Although AMD can cause permanent vision loss, patients with AMD should be encouraged to maximize the vision they have to perform activities of daily living. Low vision aids can be extremely useful to AMD patients in helping to performing activities of daily living (Table 3). Low vision professionals are experts trained at assessing remaining vision, recommending visual devices and aids, and providing training in the use of these devices.

Other helpful nonoptical aids exist and include:

- Reading stands;
- Large print publications;
- Special dials with large lettering for stoves;
- Large numbered alarm clocks;
- Audio watches that announce time; and

Table 3
Low vision aids

Devices	Description
Near vision	
Magnifiers	Both handheld and stand magnifiers are available for those individuals with unsteady hands or prefer to be hands free.
High-power reading glasses	Glasses that provide additional magnification for reading.
Telescope-mounted glasses	Miniature telescopes mounted on glasses that help to focus at near.
Closed circuit television	Letter size is magnified. In addition, letter color and background can be changed.
Adjustable lamps	Improved lighting can enhance visualization.
Distant vision	
Hand-held telescope	Hand-held telescope that focuses for distance.
Telescope mounted glasses	Miniature telescopes mounted on glasses that help to focus at distance.
Filters glasses and special lenses	Special filters and lenses can improve contrast and reduce glare.

- Cut-out stencils for writing checks and envelopes.

In the bathroom, various things can be done to improve function for patients with low vision. For example:

- Keep all bathroom cabinets closed.
- Use a wall-mounted soap dispenser.
- A wall-mounted mirror with an extension arm for shaving or applying makeup.
- Organize and alphabetize items in the medicine cabinet.
- Mark the position on the hot and cold faucet so the same temperature setting can be selected each time.
- Mark the position of the water level in the bathtub with black tape to prevent overfilling.
- Keep shampoo and other items in easily identifiable, differently shaped bottles so confusion is minimized.

SELF-MANAGEMENT STRATEGIES
Diet

Eating a diet rich in antioxidants is important in the self-management of AMD (**Table 4**).[31] One observational study found that patients with AMD with high dietary intake of green leafy vegetables such as spinach and kale had a lesser risk of developing wet AMD.[31]

Amsler Grid

Patients with dry AMD are at risk for development of the neovascular form of the disease. Approximately 2% of patients with dry AMD develop wet AMD annually.[10,19] If a patient has wet AMD in 1 eye, the incidence of developing wet AMD in the fellow eye can range from 10% to 75% over 5 years, depending on the retinal characteristics.[19,32] The earlier wet AMD can be detected and treated, the better the result for vision.[16]

The Amsler grid is a useful self-monitoring method for detecting changes in vision and progression of AMD (**Fig. 10**).[33] The patient holds the grid at a distance of

Table 4	
Dietary sources of antioxidants	
Antioxidant	**Dietary Sources**
Lutein	Kale, spinach, yellow corn, egg yolk, kiwi fruit, grapes, orange juice, zucchini, squash
Zeaxanthin	Orange pepper, kiwi fruit, grapes, spinach, orange juice, zucchini, squash
β-Carotene	Sweet potato, carrots, spinach, kale, mustard greens, collard greens, turnip greens, romaine lettuce, squash, cantaloupe melon, sweet peppers, dried apricots, peaches, prunes, peas, broccoli
Vitamin C	Cantaloupe, oranges, grapefruit, kiwi fruit, mango, papaya, pineapple, strawberries, raspberries, blueberries, cranberries, watermelon, broccoli, Brussel sprouts, cauliflower, green and red peppers, spinach, cabbage, turnip greens, tomatoes, winter squash, fortified cereals
Vitamin E	Tofu, spinach, almonds, sunflower seeds, avocados, shellfish, fish (rainbow trout, swordfish, herring, salmon), olive oil, broccoli, squash, pumpkin
Zinc	Beef, lamb, sesame seeds, pumpkin seeds, lentils, garbanzo beans, cashews, turkey, shrimp
Omega-3 fatty acids	Flaxseeds, walnuts, sardines, salmon, beef, soybeans, tofu, shrimp, Brussel sprouts, cauliflower

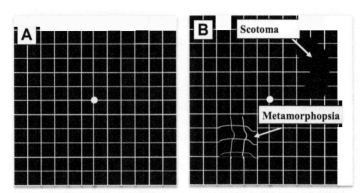

Fig. 10. The Amsler grid is a useful method of monitoring vision in patients with age-related macular degeneration. (*A*) When the grid is viewed, the horizontal and vertical lines should appear straight. (*B*) Straight lines that seem to be wavy (metamorphopsia) or absent (scotoma) are abnormalities that can be detected by the grid. If this is a new finding for the patient, the patient should notify their ophthalmologist immediately so an examination can be performed.

1 foot. The patient then covers 1 eye and focuses on the center dot with the other eye. The patient then repeats the process with the other eye. If any of the lines seem to be missing (scotoma) or wavy (metamorphopsia) and this is new for the patient, the patient should call his or her eye doctor immediately. The patient should perform this test daily at home.

ForSEEHome Device

The ForSeeHome Device is another method for monitoring of vision at home in patients with AMD.[34] Patients use the ForSeeHome Monitor daily from their home. In this test, the patients look at a screen where a series of targets flash and then disappear. The target appears as a dotted line with a bump in the line. Using a computer mouse, the patient clicks where they see the distortion. The test results are then sent immediately to the Notal Vision Data Monitoring Center. If there is a change, Notal Vision notifies the patient's eye doctor so that an eye examination can be scheduled immediately. Of the patients who used this device and converted to wet AMD, 94% kept functional vision compared with 62% who used other detection methods such as the Amsler grid.[34]

Comanagement Goals: Evaluation, Adjustment, Recurrence

Approximately, 2% of dry AMD patients will develop wet AMD every year.[10,19] Patients with wet AMD in 1 eye have a 10% to 75% risk of developing wet AMD in the fellow eye depending on the presence of high risk features.[19,32] Patients with inactive wet AMD in which treatments are stopped are also at risk for developing a recurrence of the wet AMD. Therefore, once a patient is diagnosed with AMD, they require follow-up at regular intervals with their eye care provider.

SUMMARY

AMD is the leading cause of vision loss in the elderly. The condition is diagnosed based on characteristic retinal findings. Patients with intermediate or advanced AMD should take AREDS vitamin supplements to slow down the progression of vision loss. Wet AMD can be treated with intravitreal anti-VEGF injections. Early detection and treatment of Wet AMD is important factor in retaining good and functional vision.

Amsler grid monitoring daily at home is important for individuals with AMD to help detect vision changes.

REFERENCES

1. Klein R, Rowland ML, Harris MI. Racial/ethnic differences in age-related maculopathy. Third National Health and Nutrition Examination Survey. Ophthalmology 1995;102:371–81.
2. U.S. age-specific prevalence rates for AMD by age, and race/ethnicity. 2010. Available at: https://nei.nih.gov/eyedata/amd. Accessed January 3, 2015.
3. The Eye Diseases Research Prevalence Research Group. The prevalence of diabetic retinopathy among adults in the United States. Arch Ophthalmol 2004;122:552–63.
4. Seddon JM. Epidemiology of age-related macular degeneration. In: Schachat AP, Ryan S, editors. Retina. 3rd edition. St Louis (MO): Mosby; 2001. p. 1039–50.
5. Thornton J, Edwards R, Mitchell P, et al. Smoking and age-related macular degeneration: a review of association. Eye 2005;19:935–44.
6. Van Leeuwen R, Boekhoom S, Vingerling JR, et al. Dietary intake of antioxidants and risk of age-related macular degeneration. JAMA 2005;294:3101–7.
7. Sui GY, Liu GC, Liu GY, et al. Is sunlight exposure a risk factor for age-related macular degeneration? A systematic review and meta-analysis. Br J Ophthalmol 2013;97:389–94.
8. Bhutto I, Lutty G. Understanding age-related macular degeneration (AMD): relationships between the photoreceptor/retinal pigment epithelium/Bruch's membrane/choriocapillaris complex. Mol Aspects Med 2012;33:295–317.
9. Kozlowski MR. RPE cell senescence: a key contributor to age-related macular degeneration. Med Hypotheses 2012;78:505–10.
10. The Age-Related Eye Disease Study Research Group. A randomized, placebo controlled, clinical trial of high-dose supplementation with vitamins C and E, beta carotene, and zinc for age-related macular degeneration and vision loss. AREDS Report No. 8. Arch Ophthalmol 2001;119:1417–36.
11. Holz FG, Steinberg JS, Gobel A, et al. Fundus autofluorescence imaging in dry AMD: 2014 Jules Gonin lecture of the Retina Research Foundation. Graefes Arch Clin Exp Ophthalmol 2015;253:7–16.
12. Klein R, Klein BE, Wong TY, et al. The association of cataract and cataract surgery with the long-term incidence of age-related maculopathy: the Beaver Dam Eye Study. Arch Ophthalmol 2002;120:1551–8.
13. Forooghian F, Argon E, Clemons TE, et al, Age-Related Eye Disease Study Research Group. Visual acuity outcomes after cataract surgery in patients with age-related macular degeneration: age-related eye disease study report no. 27. Ophthalmology 2009;116:2093–100.
14. Tomi A, Moldoveanu A, Marin I. Therapeutic approach in patients with age-related macular degeneration and cataract. Oftalmologia 2011;55:54–9.
15. Zlateva GP, Javitt JC, Shah SN, et al. Comparison of comorbid conditions between neovascular age-related macular degeneration patients and a control cohort in the Medicare population. Retina 2007;27:1292–9.
16. Boyer DS, Antoszyk AN, Awh CC, et al. Subgroup analysis of the MARINA study of ranibizumab in neovascular age-related macular degeneration. Ophthalmology 2007;114:246–52.
17. US Preventative Services Task Force. Screening for visual impairment. Guide to clinical preventative services. 2nd edition. Baltimore (MD): Williams & Wilkins; 1996. p. 373–82.

18. American Academy of Family Physicians. AAFP reference manual: selected policies on health issues, clinical policies, in-house (operational) policies. 1999–2000. Kansas City (MO): The American Academy of Family Physicians; 1999. p. 213.
19. AAO Retina/Vitreous PPP Panel, Hoskins Center for Quality Eye Care. American Academy of Ophthalmology preferred practice patterns for age-related macular degeneration. Available at: http://www.aao.org/preferred-practice-pattern/age-related-macular-degeneration-ppp-2015. Accessed January 3, 2015.
20. AREDS2 Research Group. Lutein/zeaxanthin and omega-3 fatty acids for age-related macular degeneration. The Age-Related Eye Disease Study 2 (AREDS2) controlled randomized clinical trial. JAMA 2013;19:2005–15.
21. The effects of vitamin E beta carotene on the incidence of lung cancer and other cancers in male smokers. The Alpha-Tocopherol, Beta Carotene Cancer Prevention Study Group. N Engl J Med 1994;330:1029–35.
22. Grisanti S, Ziemssen F. Bevacizumab: off-label use in ophthalmology. Indian J Ophthalmol 2007;55:417–20.
23. Rosenfeld PJ, Brown DM, Heier JS, et al, MARINA Study Group. Ranibizumab for neovascular age-related macular degeneration. N Engl J Med 2006;355:1419–31.
24. Comparison of Age-related Macular Degeneration Treatments Trials (CATT) Research Group, Martin DF, Maguire MG, et al. Ranibizumab and bevacizumab for treatment of neovascular age-related macular degeneration: two-year results. Ophthalmology 2012;119:1288–98.
25. Chakravarthy U, Harding SP, Rogers CA, et al, IVAN Study Investigators. Alternative treatments to inhibit VEGF in age-related choroidal neovascularization: 2 year findings of the IVAN randomized controlled trial. Lancet 2013;382:1258–67.
26. Heier JS, Brown DM, Chong V, VIEW Study Group. Intravitreal aflibercept (VEGF trap-eye) in wet age-related macular degeneration. Ophthalmology 2012;119:2537–48.
27. Schmidt-Erfurth U, Kaiser PK, Korobelnik JF, VIEW Study Group. Intravitreal aflibercept injection for neovascular age-related macular degeneration: nine-six week results of the VIEW studies. Ophthalmology 2014;121:193–201.
28. Macular Photocoagulation Study Group. Laser photocoagulation for juxtafoveal choroidal neovascularization. Five-year results from randomized clinical trials. Macular Photocoagulation Study Group. Arch Ophthalmol 1994;112:500–9.
29. Macular Photocoagulation Study Group. Laser photocoagulation for subfoveal neovascular lesions of age-related macular degeneration. Updated findings from two clinical trials. Macular Photocoagulation Study Group. Arch Ophthalmol 1993;111:1200–9.
30. Treatment of Age-Related Macular Degeneration with Photodynamic Therapy (TAP) Study Group. Photodynamic therapy of subfoveal choroidal neovascularization in age-related macular degeneration with verteporfin: one-year results of 2 randomized clinical trials—TAP report. Arch Ophthalmol 1999;117:1329–45.
31. Seddon JM, Ajani UA, Sperduto RD, et al, Eye Disease Case Control Study Group. Dietary carotenoids, vitamins A, C, and E, and advanced age-related macular degeneration. JAMA 1994;272:1413–20.
32. Wong T, Chakravarthy U, Klein R, et al. The natural history and prognosis of neovascular age-related macular degeneration: a systematic review of the literature and meta-analysis. Ophthalmology 2008;115:116–26.
33. Faes L, Bodmer NS, Bachmann LM, et al. Diagnostic accuracy of the Amsler grid and preferential hyperacuity perimetry in the screening of patients with

age-related macular degeneration: systematic review and meta-analysis. Eye 2014;28:788–96.

34. Chew EY, Clemons TE, Bressler SB, et al, The AREDS2-HOME Study Research Group. Randomized trial of a home monitoring system for early detection of choroidal neovascularization Home Monitoring of the Eye (HOME) study. Ophthalmology 2014;121:535–44.

Strabismus

Kammi B. Gunton, MD*, Barry N. Wasserman, MD,
Caroline DeBenedictis, MD

KEYWORDS

- Strabismus • Esotropia • Exotropia • Cranial nerve palsies

KEY POINTS

- Defining the type of strabismus creates a framework for work-up and management.
- Comitant esotropia is most commonly a childhood condition treated with glasses and surgery.
- Comitant exotropia is often a childhood condition that does require surgical correction.
- Microvascular disease is the most common cause of ocular cranial nerve palsies in adult patients.

INTRODUCTION

Patients with misaligned eyes often first present to a primary care clinician for evaluation. The misalignment may be intermittently present or subtle in character, making evaluation difficult. Strabismus is any misalignment of the visual axes and may be referred to as *squint*. A basic understanding of varying types of strabismus allows better communication with patients and parents as well as direct referral and treatment. Although strabismus may be referred to as *lazy eye*, the term is used in multiple diseases, such as amblyopia (decreased vision in an eye without signs of physical defect or pathology), ptosis, and strabismus. Strabismus affects 1% to 3% of children. It is seen more commonly in children with a history of prematurity; systemic diseases, such as cerebral palsy; genetic syndromes; and a family history of strabismus.[1]

Parents are often convinced that their child has a single eye that is weak, but most commonly 1 eye is simply the dominant, or fixating, eye. If the deviated eye is forced to fixate by covering the dominant eye momentarily, however, then the deviation seems to switch eyes. This demonstrates that the neuromuscular imbalance is between the eyes and is usually not limited to 1 eye or the other. In patients with palsy of a cranial nerve or 1 muscle, the dominant eye continues to fixate even if it has the effected muscle.[2]

Department of Pediatric Ophthalmology, Wills Eye Hospital, 840 Walnut Street, Suite 1210, Philadelphia, PA, USA
* Corresponding author.
E-mail address: kbgunton@comcast.net

Prim Care Clin Office Pract 42 (2015) 393–407
http://dx.doi.org/10.1016/j.pop.2015.05.006   **primarycare.theclinics.com**

The most common form of strabismus is in the horizontal axis. An eye crossed relative to the other is called an esotropia, whereas an outward drift of 1 eye is called an exotropia. In vertical deviations, the effected eye must be specified, because a left hypertropia is the same as a right hypotropia. More complex forms of strabismus have differing misalignment in various gazes. Deviations are further defined by their comitance. Comitant deviations are the same in all directions of gaze, and incomitant deviations vary depending on the gaze. Nevertheless, the basic approach to strabismus includes defining the type of strabismus, recognizing patterns of misalignment, and applying the appropriate work-up/treatment. This review covers the basic types of comitant esotropia and exotropia and misalignments seen in cranial nerve palsies. Special syndromes and systemic diseases that directly affect the extraocular muscles and restrictive processes are beyond the scope of this review.

Assessment of strabismus is performed by several different techniques. Various basic techniques are excellent for screening patients. The Hirschberg method involves shining a beam of light at the eyes and assessing the light reflex in the pupils. If the eyes are aligned, then the light is essentially centered within the pupil. If a child is looking directly at the light, and 1 light reflex is in the center of the pupil and the other light reflex is not, then strabismus is suspected. Another useful technique is the Bruckner technique. With the room lights dimmed and standing a few feet from the patient, the clinician holds the direct ophthalmoscope to his or her eye and directs the instrument light toward the child's face. The red reflex should be seen equally. If there is asymmetry of the red reflex, strabismus or other ocular pathology should be suspected. If the child is old enough to hold attention with a toy, then a cover test can be attempted. With the toy in front of the child, 1 eye is briefly covered while observing the motion of the uncovered eye. If the uncovered eye moves to find the toy, then strabismus is present. If there is no strabismus, then no refixation movement of either eye should be seen. The appropriate technique used depends on the comfort level of the clinician and the cooperation of the patient. Ultimately, if strabismus is manifest a majority of the time, the child loses binocularity and could become amblyopic. Adults with strabismus may have disabling diplopia.

ESOTROPIA

Esotropia is a type of ocular misalignment in which the deviating eye turns in medially, toward the nose (**Fig. 1**). In the first months of life, the visual and oculomotor systems are immature and still developing. Parents may think their child's eyes are crossed or drifting out, but the duration of the misalignment is generally brief, and realignment is established spontaneously. The eyes should achieve stable alignment for most

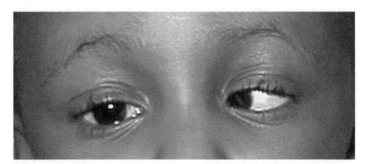

Fig. 1. Esotropia (crossing) of left eye. (*Courtesy of* Kammi B. Gunton, MD.)

children by 3 months but can be delayed in children who are premature or those with delayed visual maturation. If there is suspicion of ocular misalignment beyond 3 months of age, then referral to a pediatric ophthalmologist should be considered. There are several types of comitant esotropia. The most common types—pseudoesotropia, congenital esotropia, and accommodative esotropia—are discussed.

Pseudoesotropia

Pseudoesotropia represents a large portion of the consultations in a pediatric ophthalmology practice.[3] The term *pseudo* implies a false esotropia. The ocular alignment is normal, but the appearance of the eyes suggests crossing. Infants often have wide nasal bridges and prominent epicanthal folds. A prominent epicanthal fold covers the medial sclera of both eyes, making the eyes appear crossed. Referral to an ophthalmologist to verify the alignment is appropriate. Treatment consists of an explanation of the cause of the appearance of crossing with reassurance to parents that true crossing is not present and observation because some children have pseudoesotropia initially but later develop intermittent esotropia. Repeat examinations on separate visits may reveal true strabismus.

Congenital Esotropia

Congenital esotropia is an ocular misalignment with onset in the first 6 months of life. Any child with constant crossing of the eyes should be referred to the ophthalmologist at presentation. Only small-angle, intermittent crossing can be observed in the first 3 months of life, because it may spontaneously resolve. In congenital esotropia, the angle of deviation is usually large, and patients may switch the fixating eye spontaneously (**Fig. 2**). Patients typically have no significant refractive error.[4,5] Several other ocular findings may be seen in these patients. They may have latent nystagmus, a shaking or jiggling of the eye when 1 eye is covered. They may have oblique eye muscle dysfunction, which can lead to pattern esotropia. For example, a V-pattern esotropia is associated with inferior oblique muscle dysfunction and has a much larger angle of deviation in downgaze with a smaller angle of deviation in upgaze. Dissociated vertical deviations also are seen in association with congenital esotropia and involve a unilateral upward drift of the nonfixing eye. Treatment of congenital esotropia is surgical.[4,6] Glasses are rarely helpful, and there is no role for eye exercises, commonly called vision therapy.

Accommodative Esotropia

Accommodative esotropia generally occurs between 1 and 3 years of age.[7,8] This type of esotropia is associated with high hyperopic (farsighted) refractive errors. Most children in this age group are naturally mildly hyperopic, but young people can accommodate or adjust their focus. They have no particular trouble with their sight for distance or near targets. The near reflex, however, includes convergence with accommodation.

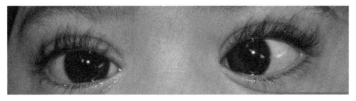

Fig. 2. Congenital esotropia (crossing) with right eye fixing on target. (*Courtesy of* Barry N. Wasserman, MD.)

When children with accommodative esotropia with large amounts of hyperopia accommodate, they converge and are unable to perform a fusional divergence movement, which would realign the visual axis. An esotropia results (**Fig. 3**). Fortunately, correction with hyperopic spectacles relaxes the accommodation and its associated esotropia. In some patients, excessive convergence for accommodation results in further crossing of the eyes when viewing near targets. This is referred to as a high accommodative convergence to accommodation ratio. In these patients, a bifocal lens further relaxes accommodation at near-target fixation and alleviates the residual esotropia through the bifocal. Once acceptable ocular alignment is achieved in patients with accommodative esotropia, they may still require treatment of amblyopia (poor vision in nonpreferred eye). Hyperopia classically diminishes with development into adolescence. If treatment is delayed, residual esotropia despite spectacle correction remains. In these cases, strabismus surgery can achieve excellent ocular alignment.[7] Early referral to an ophthalmologist for treatment with glasses can prevent the need for surgery and amblyopia treatment.

The acute onset of comitant esotropia in older children can have a neurologic basis. Children over 5 years old often complain of acute diplopia (double vision). In the absence of refractive error, this type of esotropia may be associated with intracranial pathology, including Arnold-Chiari type I malformation, pontine gliomas, and astrocytomas.[8] Urgent neuroimaging is indicated, as is immediate referral.

EXODEVIATIONS

An exodeviation is the outward drift of 1 eye compared with the other (**Fig. 4**). There are several types of exodeviations, including pseudoexotropia, exophoria, intermittent exotropia, constant exotropia, and convergence insufficiency. In all cases, parental observations of the frequency of the misalignment and eye preference should be elicited. A medical history of craniofacial syndromes, neurologic disorders, infections, and trauma may predispose to exodeviations. Specific genes have not yet been identified, but there is often a family history of exotropia.

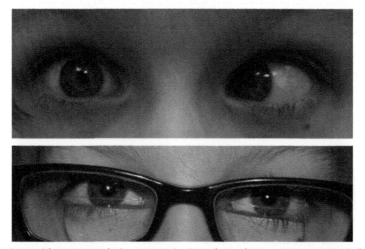

Fig. 3. Patient with accommodative esotropia. Top photo demonstrates esotropia (crossing) of the left eye without spectacle correction. Bottom photo of same patient with aligned eyes in glasses. (*Courtesy of* Barry N. Wasserman, MD.)

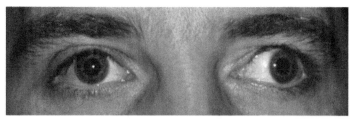

Fig. 4. Exotropia (outward drift) with right eye fixing. (*Courtesy of* Kammi B. Gunton, MD.)

Pseudoexotropia

Pseudoexotropia occurs when the globes are properly aligned but the eyes have the appearance of outward divergence. This can result from a wide interpupillary distance or a positive angle kappa. Angle kappa is the angle formed between the visual and pupillary axes. If the angle between these 2 axes is larger than 5°, the corneal light reflex is nasally displaced, forming a positive angle kappa. This gives the appearance of an exotropia. Positive angle kappa can occur in isolation or as a result of intraocular abnormalities, including temporal macular dragging caused by retinopathy of prematurity, high myopia, or infection with macular scarring. Children with pseudoexotropia maintain a straight head position, and there is no refixation movement with cover testing. No treatment of the alignment is required, but amblyopia accompanying the macular pathology must be addressed if applicable.

Exophoria

An exodeviation that is controlled by the sensory fusional mechanisms of binocular vision is called an exophoria. Under normal viewing conditions, the eyes are in proper alignment. If binocular fusion is disrupted, however, the exodeviation emerges. In the absence of symptoms, no treatment is indicated. Observation is recommended because decompensation results in progression to manifest exotropia.

Intermittent Exotropia

Intermittent exotropia is the most common form of exodeviation in childhood. The age of onset is variable but generally occurs between 6 months and 4 years of age. The exodeviation is intermittently present. Initially, the deviation occurs with periods of inattention, fatigue, and stress. Parents may note intermittent squinting or children closing 1 eye, especially in bright light. This behavior occurs to prevent diplopia when the eye is exotropic. Bright light often disrupts fusion, allowing the exodeviation to become manifest. Additionally, the eyes may realign with near fixation, deviating only when the patient looks off into the distance. With progression, the deviation may occur with near viewing. The periods of misalignment may become more frequent and progress to constant exotropia. Patients typically have good vision in both eyes without amblyopia and may alternate the fixing eye.

Intermittent exotropia is divided into 3 classifications. Basic exotropia is characterized by an exodeviation that measures the same at distance and at near. Divergence excess is an exodeviation greater at distance than near. Lastly, convergence insufficiency exotropia is an exodeviation greater at near than at distance.

Less invasive treatments are preferred to surgical intervention if possible. Preservation of vision, binocular fusion, and proper alignment drive the treatment of exodeviations. Treatment begins by correcting any underlying pathology. Significant refractive errors should be corrected with glasses. Any amblyopia must be treated with glasses and/or patching. Prisms are an option for small deviations that cause diplopia, although they are usually reserved as a treatment in adult-onset exotropia or patients who are not surgical candidates. Vision therapy alone has not proved to effectively treat exotropia.[9] In cases of extremely large, frequent, or constant exotropia, surgical intervention may be undertaken. The timing of surgery is variable. Most surgeons wait until the exotropia occurs at least 50% of the waking hours and measures greater than 14 to 16 prism diopters (PD). Surgery is undertaken earlier if the exodeviation causes amblyopia or significantly effects binocular fusion. Surgical options include bilateral lateral rectus recessions or unilateral recession of lateral rectus with resection of medial rectus. Although both procedures provide good results with initial alignment, long-term success is harder to define.[10] The most common complications of strabismus surgery include overcorrection, undercorrection, or recurrent strabismus after a period of realignment.

Constant Exotropia

Constant exotropia occurs when the eyes are constantly deviated. It is more common in older patients or in patients with decompensated intermittent exotropia, although a congenital type exists. There are different classifications of constant exotropia.

Congenital exotropia occurs before the age of 6 months to 1 year. This is a rare form of exotropia in healthy children. It is more common in children with neurologic disease or craniofacial disorders. It can begin as an intermittent deviation but rapidly progresses to a constant exotropia. As in congenital esotropia, the angle of deviation in congenital exotropia is large, usually more than 35 PDs. These children are typically treated with early surgery to try to regain some binocularity. They should be followed closely during the amblyogenic years to monitor the vision and new misalignments, such as vertical deviations or esotropia.

Sensory exotropia is typically a unilateral exodeviation occurring in patients with significantly reduced visual acuity in 1 eye. Potential causes include anisometropic amblyopia, corneal opacities, cataracts, optic nerve hypoplasia or atrophy, and retinal pathology. The eye with poor vision become strabismic. It can be esotropic or exotropic, with exotropia occurring more commonly in older children and adults. Consecutive exotropia occurs after previous strabismus surgery for esotropia and recurrent exotropia follows previous surgery for exotropia. These deviations occur in patients with poor binocularity. Surgical treatment is required to realign the eyes, but gradual misalignment likely recurs.

Convergence Insufficiency

Convergence insufficiency is defined as an exophoria that is greater at near than at distance. Characteristics include asthenopia with near vision, blurred near vision, reading problems, decreased near point of convergence, and decreased near fusional convergence amplitudes. The options for treatment include vision therapy exercises or prism glasses. Vision therapy is effective in convergence insufficiency.[11] Prismatic correction in reading glasses may also provide relief of symptoms.

OCULAR CRANIAL NERVE PALSIES

The 6 extraocular muscles are responsible for the coordinated motility of the eyes. They are supplied by 3 cranial nerves. Diseases effecting any of the nerves, therefore, result in a particular pattern of motility disturbance. Cranial nerve palsies may result in complete or partial weakness of the corresponding muscles. In reviews of cranial nerve palsies, women and men seem equally effected, and 38% of patients have associated systemic disease.[12] Sixth nerve palsies are the most common of the 3, accounting for 58%[13] of cases; followed by third nerve palsies, 26% percent of cases; and fourth nerve palsies, 16% percent of all cases. The motility patterns caused by cranial nerve palsies, their causes, work-up, and finally treatment options are reviewed.

Sixth Cranial Nerve

The sixth cranial nerve or the abducens nerve supplies the ipsilateral lateral rectus muscle, which is responsible for abduction of the eye. Therefore, the pattern of strabismus that results from palsy is an esotropia worse in gaze to the effected side (**Fig. 5**). Patients often adopt a face turn away from the eye with the palsied muscle to restore binocularity or report horizontal diplopia in side gaze depending on the complete or partial nature of the palsy.

The abducens nerve originates in the pons and ascends to coordinate side gaze with fibers in the contralateral medial rectus. Gaze palsy, therefore, results from lesions within the abducens nucleus. Nuclear palsies can occur from pontine infarctions or gliomas, cerebellar tumors, and alcoholic encephalopathy. The abducens nerve exits the pons adjacent to the V, VII, and VIII nerves. Therefore, damage to the

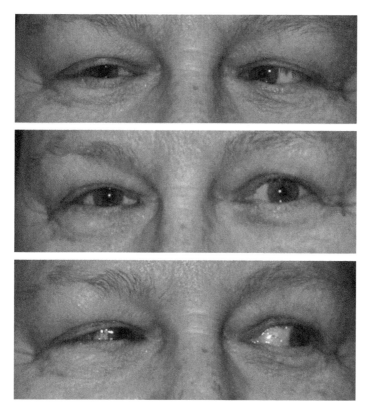

Fig. 5. Sixth nerve palsy right eye. Top photo reveals lack of abduction of right eye. Middle phots shows right face turn to achieve binocularity in primary position. Bottom photo shows normal left gaze. (*Courtesy of* Kammi B. Gunton, MD.)

fasciculus results in ipsilateral abduction weakness accompanied by ipsilateral facial weakness and analgesia, ipsilateral Horner, and ipsilateral deafness. The cause of fascicular palsies is most often vascular disease.

The abducens nerve then climbs along the clivus, making it vulnerable to compressive lesions by basilar tumors, such as acoustic neuromas, nasopharyngeal carcinomas, and menigiomas. In addition, elevated intracranial pressure resulting in downward displacement of the brainstem stretches the abducens nerve at this location. Once the nerve pierces the dura, it travels around the inferior petrosal sinus, making it susceptible to trauma of the temporal bone or infections of the mastoid.

Congenital lesions of the sixth nerve are rare. Etiology of sixth nerve palsies falls into 5 broad categories: idiopathic, 8% to 30%; tumors and other miscellaneous, 10% to 30%; traumatic, 3% to 30%; and vascular causes, 0% to 36%.[14–17] In adults over 50 years of age, the most common cause is microvascular disease and spontaneous resolution is common.[14,18] In elderly patients, giant cell arteritis must be considered. Without vasculopathic risk factors, neuroimaging, lumbar puncture, and blood work, including complete blood cell count (CBC), sedimentation rate, Lyme disease, and syphilis testing, may be indicated (**Table 1**).

The work-up of sixth nerve palsy depends on the age and accompanying general health of the patient. In children, an aggressive work-up is warranted. In 1 series of children with isolated sixth nerve palsy without papilledema or known cranial

Table 1
Work-up strategies for ocular cranial nerve palsies

Cranial Nerve Palsies	Oculomotor, III	Trochlear, IV	Abducens, VI
Vasculopathic age group, with isolated nerve palsy	Pupil sparing: observe for 5 d to rule out pupil involvement. Check blood pressure, fasting blood sugar and other parameters of diabetic control, cholesterol levels. In patients >65, test for giant cell arteritis.[14–17] Pupil involving: emergent MRA/cerebral angiogram for aneurysms[18]	Check blood pressure, fasting blood sugar and other parameters of diabetic control, and cholesterol levels.	Check blood pressure, fasting blood sugar and other parameters of diabetic control, and cholesterol levels. In patients >65, test for giant cell arteritis.
Nonresolving, or younger patients	MRI/MRA with contrast, CBC with differential, sedimentation rate, tests for myasthenia[14–16]	MRI with contrast, CBC with differential, tests for myasthenia, fasting blood sugar	MRI with contrast focusing on pathway of VI nerve and increased intracranial pressure, CBC with differential, sedimentation rate, Lyme disease antibodies, syphilis, thyroid testing, tests for myasthenia gravis

Data from Refs.[14–16]

pathology, tumor was found in 31% of patients.[19] Any associated signs, such as Horner, other cranial nerve involvement, nystagmus, papilledema, and contralateral weakness, necessitate neuroimaging with MRI to assess the brainstem. In addition, elevated intracranial pressure from any cause, including idiopathic intracranial hypertension (IIH), may result in unilateral or bilateral sixth nerve palsies in as many as 60% of cases.[20] Sixth nerve palsies may also occur as postviral syndromes or in association with multiple sclerosis.

Microvascular causes secondary to hypertension or diabetes resolve spontaneously over a 6- to 12-month period. Spontaneous resolution occurs in approximately 66% to 73% of patients.[14,18] Traumatic causes resolve in 27% to 50% of cases.[21] Lack of improvement of symptoms warrants a more aggressive work-up if microvascular disease were initially suspected. Patching relieves the diplopia associated with sixth nerve palsies. In children less than 8 years of age who are vulnerable to amblyopia, alternate eye patching is indicated. Prism may also relieve the symptoms in primary position, but diplopia is still likely in side gazes. Treatment is otherwise tailored to the cause. With idiopathic etiology or nonresolving microvascular disease after 6 months, surgery to weaken the ipsilateral medial rectus, strengthen the ipsilateral lateral rectus, or transpose the ipsilateral superior rectus or both superior and inferior rectus to the lateral rectus may be indicated depending on the extent of the palsy.[22,23] Approximately 80% of patients in 1 series achieved an acceptable range of single vision after surgery.[18]

Third Cranial Nerve

The third cranial nerve controls 4 of the 6 extraocular muscles. The nerve divides when entering into the orbit into superior and inferior divisions. The superior division controls the superior rectus and the levator palpebrae whereas the inferior division controls the medial rectus, inferior rectus, and inferior oblique. The pupillary constrictor fibers travel with the inferior division as well. Therefore, complete or partial palsies of the oculomotor nerve can present with a variety of deviations. Complete palsies are more easily recognized with complete ptosis, pupillary dilation, exotropia, and depression of the globe (**Fig. 6**). Diplopia may initially be masked due to the ptosis. Pupillary dilation can cause light sensitivity and poor accommodation. Incomplete palsies present with signs and symptoms particular to the muscles effected.

The oculomotor nucleus is complex nucleus with multiple subnuclei in the brainstem. The fibers innervating the levator palpebrae are shared by a single midline subnucleus. The fibers to the superior rectus are unique in that they cross on leaving the nucleus. Therefore, lesions within the oculomotor nerve nucleus can lead to bilateral ptosis and contralateral limitations in elevation. Associated tremors or spastic paralysis implies a nuclear or fascicular lesion, which requires MRI to elucidate.

Within the subarachnoid space, the peripheral nerve is vulnerable to aneurysms of the posterior communicating artery. Acute presentation of an oculomotor palsy with pupillary involvement requires magnetic resonance angiogram (MRA)/arteriography imaging to rule out this life-threatening aneurysm. Uncal herniation and trauma can also effect the nerve as it pierces the dura. Pupillary fibers are effected first when palsy occurs from a traumatic cause, because the pupillary fibers are more superficial and located dorsal-medially within the nerve at this location.

In the cavernous sinus, the oculomotor nerve travels in the lateral dorsal wall adjacent to the fourth nerve. Cavernous sinus fistulas, aneurysms, tumors, pituitary apoplexy, and infections/inflammations within the cavernous sinus can present with accompanying palsy of any of the ocular cranial nerves.

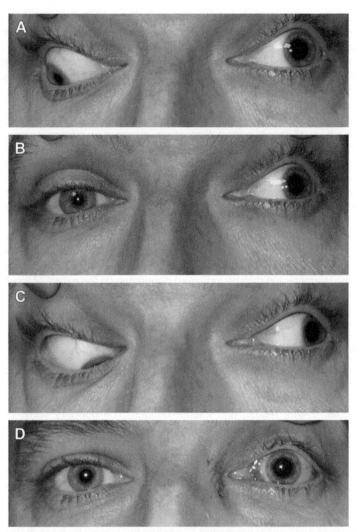

Fig. 6. Third nerve palsy left eye. (*A*) Inability to adduct the left eye to midline. (*B*) Dilated pupil with exotropia (outward drift) of left eye in primary position. (*C*) Normal abduction with limited depression of left eye. (*D*) Same patient with eyes in primary position post–left globe fixation surgery. (*Courtesy of* Kammi B. Gunton, MD.)

Within the orbit, trauma, local neoplastic processes and infections can effect either the superior or inferior division of the third nerve. In 1 review of head injuries, approximately half had some associated ocular morbidity and 11.6% of those patients had complete or partial oculomotor nerve palsy.[24] In addition, migraines may result in partial oculomotor palsies. Recent studies reveal that in up to one-third of cases of migraine, a demyelinating process or neuropathy is actually to blame for the nerve palsy.[25]

The most common cause of pupillary sparing oculomotor palsy is ischemia. In patients over 50 with atherosclerotic risk factors, an isolated, pupil-sparing oculomotor palsy is likely due to microvascular disease and neuroimaging is not required.[26,27]

Ischemic damage typically resolves spontaneously within 3 to 6 months. In older adults, testing for giant cell arteritis is indicated. A complete work-up includes a CBC, glucose tolerance testing, sedimentation rate, blood pressure, syphilis testing, and antinuclear antibody testing.[27] In addition, close observation of the pupil is required because evolution to pupil involvement can occur within the first 5 days of presentation. Pupillary involvement requires emergent neuroimaging with attention to aneurysms (MRI/MRA) and prompt referral to neurosurgeons (see **Table 1**).

In children, congenital causes and trauma are the most common causes of oculomotor palsies.[27] Yet, in 1 series from Nigeria of young patients aged 20 to 29 years, systemic disorders were found in 38% of patients presenting with cranial nerve palsy.[12] Other causes of oculomotor palsy that are not localizing include migraines; myasthenia; postvaccination inflammation; granulomatous diseases, such as sarcoid; meningitis from infectious causes; IIH; and multiple sclerosis.[12,25,28–30]

Spontaneous recovery of the third nerve can result in misdirection of the nerve fibers into other muscles supplied by the third nerve. This is known as aberrant regeneration. The most common misdirections are elevation of the upper eyelid with adduction or depression of the eye, adduction of the eye on attempted downgaze, and segmental pupillary constriction with adduction. Aberrant regeneration occurs with recovery from trauma, aneurysm or tumors but not from microvascular insults, such as from diabetic disease. Presence of aberrant regeneration should redirect a work-up to these other causes.

Treatment of oculomotor palsy is directed toward the underlying causes if possible. Six months after presentation of symptoms, strabismus surgery may be recommended if recovery is incomplete from microvascular cause. Treatment focuses on managing the symptoms in primary position and incorporating the complexity of the misalignment present. If an acceptable range of single vision cannot be achieved, occlusion of 1 eye is a reasonable alternative. Possible surgical alternatives include globe fixation procedures with various suture materials, disinsertion of the lateral rectus, and/or superior oblique or transpositions of these muscles to allow centration of the globe.[30] Preoperative assessment of any residual function within the muscles supplied by the oculomotor nerve also has an impact on surgical choices.

Fourth Cranial Nerve

The fourth cranial nerve, or trochlear nerve supplies the superior oblique muscle. The superior oblique muscle's primary function is to intort, or rotate the eye toward the nose. This cycloduction movement occurs when the head is tilted to the side. To maintain stability of the visual field, the eyes perform a counter-rotation to the head. For example, if the head tilts to the right shoulder, the right eye intorts and the left eye extorts, or rotates toward the ear. The superior rectus muscle also acts as an agonist to intort the eye. In cases of superior oblique palsy, the elevation occurring due to superior rectus activity cannot be countered by the superior oblique when intorting the eye, and a hyperdeviation results when tilting the head toward the side of the palsied eye.

In addition, the superior oblique is a depressor and an abductor of the eye. With palsy of the superior oblique, a hyperdeviation results. The superior oblique has the greatest effect on the vertical position when an eye is adducted. Therefore, the degree of diplopia in a superior oblique palsy is worse in gaze away from the eye with the palsied muscle (**Fig. 7**).

The Parks 3-step test is used to identify which vertical muscle is the cause of a hyperdeviation. The first step of the test is to determine the deviation with the eyes in the primary position, which is gazing straight ahead with the head straight. A hyperdeviation in primary position indicates a weakness in the depressors of the effected

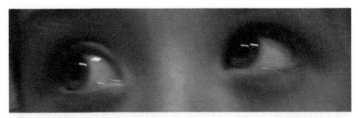

Fig. 7. Fourth nerve palsy of left eye showing hyperdeviation in adducted position. (*Courtesy of* Kammi B. Gunton, MD.)

eye or the elevators of the contralateral eye. The second step assesses which horizontal gaze worsens the deviation. The vertical rectus muscles have greater effect when an eye is abducted, and the obliques have greater vertical effect when an eye is adducted. The third step uses head tilt to determine if the deviation is worse with intorsion or extorsion. The results from the 3 steps yield the causative palsied muscle. Although the 3-step test is useful, it cannot be used in cases of restrictive processes effecting the muscles or multiple muscle palsies.[31]

Vertical and torsional diplopia may result from fourth cranial nerve palsies. Patients with congenital causes have intermittent symptoms or diplopia only in certain gazes due to adaptive vergences, whereas patients with acquired causes usually have sudden onset of constant diplopia. The ability to fuse large vertical deviations is highly suggestive of a congenital cause. Most patients also adapt a head tilt away from the side of the palsied muscle, because the vertical deviation is smaller and more easily controlled in this position. Old photographs showing the head tilt can support the long-standing nature of congenital palsies.

Acquired lesions are more often due to lesions along the course of the trochlear nerve and less frequently within the superior oblique muscle or tendon.[32,33] Causes include trauma, neoplasm, ischemia, increased intracranial pressure, aneurysm, meningitis, and idiopathic. The fourth nerve also originates in the brainstem and decussates on exiting. Vascular disease, trauma, and demyelinated processes may cause injury within the brainstem resulting in contralateral superior oblique palsy, but often accompanying symptoms occur from adjacent structures, such as the descending sympathetic fibers, which can cause a Horner syndrome ipsilaterally.

The peripheral trochlear nerve courses around the brainstem, pierces the dura, and, via the cavernous sinus, enters the superior orbital fissure. This long course makes it susceptible to closed head trauma. Ischemic injury is the second most common cause of superior oblique palsy after trauma. Inquiring about hypertension, diabetes, and other vascular ischemic risk factors is helpful. Hydrocephalus, IIH, and tumors compressing its pathway can also lead to superior oblique palsy.[20] An acquired cause, therefore, requires neuroimaging (see **Table 1**).

Ischemic superior oblique palsies usually spontaneously resolve within 6 months. Treatment, therefore, requires supportive measures until resolution. These measures include patching 1 eye, prisms within glasses to alleviate some of the symptoms, or, in cases without resolution, surgery to balance the remaining weakness. Surgical choices are guided by Knapp guidelines, which suggest surgery on the muscle acting when the deviation is at its greatest. These muscles include the ipsilateral superior oblique, inferior oblique, and superior rectus or the contralateral inferior rectus. Deviations greater than 15 PDs or 7° of vertical deviation generally require 2-muscle surgery.[34,35] Torsion can be best addressed with surgery on the superior oblique muscle.[36] Surgical success with fusion in primary position after surgical correction is greater when the preoperative deviation is smaller than 15 PDs.[37–39] Success rates vary from 60% to 65% when the deviation is larger.[34]

SUMMARY

With a systematic approach to the strabismus patient, an appropriate work-up and treatment plan may be instituted. Recognizing the type of misalignment and identifying any incomitance narrows the differential substantially. Treatment options differ by the cause and type of misalignment, and success rates also vary depending on the binocularity of the patient. Nevertheless, relieving the symptoms of asthenopia and diplopia in patients is life altering for many.

REFERENCES

1. McKean-Cowdin R, Cotter SA, Traczy-Hornoch K, et al. Prevalence of amblyopia or strabismus in Asian and non-Hispanic white preschool children: multi-ethnic pediatric eye disease study. Ophthalmol 2013;120:2117–24.
2. Simon JW, Aggarwal NK, editors. The pediatric eye examination. Philadelphia: Lippincott, Willimas and Wilkins; 2005. p. 87–91 (Nelson LB, Olitsky SE, editors. Harley's Pediatric Ophthalmology. 5th Edition).
3. Hutcheson KA. Childhood esotropia. Curr Opin Ophthalmol 2004;15:444–8.
4. Forbes BJ, Khazaeni LM. Evaluation and management of an infantile esotropia. Pediatr Case Rev 2003;3:211–4.
5. Campos EC. Why do the eyes cross? A review and discussion of the nature and origin of essential infantile esotropia, microstrabismus, accommodative esotropia, and acute comitant esotropia. J AAPOS 2008;12:326–31.
6. Gunton KB, Nelson BA. Evidence-based medicine in congenital esotropia. J Pediatr Ophthalmol Strabismus 2003;40:70–3.
7. Lambert SR. Accommodative esotropia. Ophthalmol Clin North Am 2001;14: 425–32.
8. Schworm HD, Rudolph G. Comitant strabismus. Curr Opin Ophthalmol 2000;11: 310–7.
9. Gnanaraj L, Richardson SR. Interventions for intermittent distance exotropia: review. Eye 2005;19:617–21.
10. Joyce KE, Beyer F, Thomason RG, et al. A systematic review of the effectiveness of treatments in altering the natural history of intermittent exotropia. Br J Ophthalmol 2014;99(4):440–50.
11. Scheiman M, Mitchell GL, Cotter S, et al. A randomized clinical trial of treatments for convergence insufficiency in children. Arch Ophthalmol 2005;123:14–24.
12. Pedro-Egbe CN, Fiebai B, Awoyesuku EA. A 3-year review of cranial nerve palsies from the University of Port Harcourt teaching hospital eye clinic, Nigeria. Middle East Afr J Ophthalmol 2014;21:170–4.
13. Rowe F. Prevalence of ocular motor cranial nerve palsy and associations following stroke. Eye 2011;25:881–7.
14. Richards BW, Jones FR, Younge BR, et al. Causes and prognosis in 4,278 cases of paralysis of the oculomotor, trochlear and abducens cranial nerves. Am J Ophthalmol 1992;113:489–96.
15. Peters GB, Bakri SJ, Kohel GB. Cause and prognosis of nontraumatic sixth nerve palsies in young adults. Ophthalmology 2002;109:1925–8.
16. Moster ML, Savino PJ, Sergot RC, et al. Isolated sixth-nerve palsies in young adults. Arch Ophthalmol 1984;102:1328–30.

17. Kodsi SR, Younge BR. Acquired oculomotor, trochlear, and aducent cranial nerve palsies in pediatric patients. Am J Ophthalmol 1992;114:568–74.

18. Surachatkumtonekul T, Soontrapa P, Kampanartsanyakorn S, et al. Causes and treatment outcomes of third, fourth and sixth cranial nerve palsy. J Med Assoc Thai 2012;95:S96–101.

19. Dotan G, Rosenfeld E, Stolovitch C, et al. The role of neuroimaging in the evaluation process of children with isolated sixth nerve palsy. Childs Nerv Syst 2013; 29:89–92.

20. Patton N, Beatty S, Lloyd C. Bilateral sixth and fourth cranial nerve palsies in idiopathic intracranial hypertension. J R Soc Med 2000;93:80–1.

21. Bianchi-Marzoli S, Brancato R. Third, fourth, and sixth cranial nerve palsies. Curr Opin Ophthalmol 1997;8:45–51.

22. Holmes JM, Hatt SR, Leske DA. Intraoperative monitoring of torsion to prevent vertical deviations during augmented vertical rectus transposition surgery. J AAPOS 2012;16:136–40.

23. Mehendale RA, Dagi LR, Wu C, et al. Superior rectus transposition and medial rectus recession for Duane syndrome and sixth nerve palsy. Arch Ophthalmol 2012;130:195–201.

24. Sharma B, Gupta R, Anand R, et al. Ocular manifestations of head injury and incidence of post-traumatic ocular motor nerve involvement in cases of head injury: a clinical review. Int Ophthalmol 2014;34:893–900.

25. Gelfand AA, Gelfand JM, Prabakhar P, et al. Ophthalmoplegic "migraine" or recurrent ophthalmoplegic cranial neuropathy: new cases and a systemic review. J Child Neurol 2012;27:759–66.

26. Murchison AP, Gilbert ME, Savino PJ. Nueroimaging and acute ocular motor mononeuropathies: a prospective study. Arch Ophthalmol 2011;129:301–5.

27. Yanovitch T, Buckley E. Diagnosis and management of third nerve palsy. Curr Opin Ophthalmol 2007;18:373–8.

28. Woo EJ, Winiecki SK, Ou AC. Motor palsies of cranial nerves (excluding VII) afer vaccination: reports to the US Vaccine Adverse Event Reporting System. Hum Vaccin Immunother 2014;10:301–5.

29. Muralidhar R, Vijayalakshmi P, Mahesh S, et al. Ophthalmic migraine with pupil-sparing third nerve palsy. J Pediatr Ophthalmol Strabismus 2013;50:320.

30. Sadagopan KA, Wasserman BN. Managing the patient with oculomotor nerve palsy. Curr Opin Ophthalmol 2013;24:438–47.

31. Muthusamy B, Irsch K, Chang HP, et al. The sensitivity of the Bielschowsky head-tilt test in diagnosing acquired bilateral superior oblique paresis. Am J Ophthalmol 2014;157:901–7.

32. Nelson LB. Acute fourth nerve palsy. J Pediatr Ophthalmol Strabismus 2012;49:1.

33. Merino PS, Rojas PL, Gómez De Liaño PS, et al. Bilateral superior oblique palsy: etiology and therapeutic options. Eur J Ophthalmol 2014;24:147–52.

34. Nejad M, Thacker N, Velez FG, et al. Surgical results of patients with unilateral superior oblique palsy presenting with larger hypertropia. J Pediatr Ophthalmol Strabismus 2013;50:44–52.

35. Sekeroğlu HT, Sanac AS, Arsian U, et al. Superior oblique surgery: when and how? Clin Ophthalmol 2013;7:1571–4.

36. Li Y, Zhao K. Superior oblique tucking for treatment of superior oblique palsy. J Pediatr Ophthalmol Strabismus 2014;51:249–54.

37. Mulvihill A, Murphy M, Lee JP. Disinsertion of the inferior oblique muscle for treatment of superior oblique paresis. J Pediatr Ophthalmol Strabismus 2000;37: 279–82.

38. Morad Y, Weinstock VM, Kraft SP. Outcome of inferior oblique recession with or without vertical rectus recession for unilateral superior oblique palsy. Binocul Vis Strabismus Q 2001;18(1):23–8.
39. Durnian JM, Marsh IB. Superior oblique tuck: it's success as a muscle treatment for selected cases of superior oblique palsy. Strabismus 2011;19:133–7.

Cataracts

Jay Thompson, MD[a],*, Naheed Lakhani, MD[b]

KEYWORDS

- Cataracts • Intraocular lens implant • Surgery • Management • Cataract symptoms

KEY POINTS

- A cataract is the term used to describe the opacification of the crystalline lens inside the eye.
- Primary care providers play a key role in diagnosing cataracts based on symptoms and known risk factors.
- Cataract surgery is one of the most successful of all surgical procedures performed.
- There are currently no medical treatment for cataracts, however, minimizing exposure to known risk factors can slow progression.

INTRODUCTION

A cataract is a clouding of the crystalline lens inside the eye, which leads to a decrease in vision. It is the most prevalent, treatable cause of visual impairment and blindness in the world. Cataract surgery with an intraocular lens (IOL) implant is one of the most common and thought to be the most effective surgical procedure in any field of medicine. Although aging is the most common cause, other factors, including disease, trauma, medications, and genetic predisposition, are also known to be associated with cataract formation.[1] Although cataracts, and the subsequent surgery to correct them, are ultimately the domain of ophthalmology, the primary care physician is frequently the one to whom patients present with vision complaints. Knowledge of cataract symptoms, how to evaluate them, and a basic understanding of the surgery to correct cataracts make primary care physicians an integral part of treating this leading cause of preventable blindness.

Cataract Surgery: A Brief History

Cataract surgery today is defined as the removal of the opacified lens and replacement with a synthetic lens known as an IOL. Up until the 1960s and later, the cataract was simply removed without a replacement. Although the potential of vision was restored, the resulting lack of a lens, or aphakia, resulted in a significant hyperopia caused by the absence of the lens' focusing power. Thus, in order to have focused vision it was

[a] Lowcountry Eye Specialists, 9565 Highway 78, #100, Ladson, SC 20456, USA; [b] Emory Family Medicine Residency Program, 718 Gatewood Road NE, Atlanta, GA 30322, USA
* Corresponding author.
E-mail address: jt3md@yahoo.com

Prim Care Clin Office Pract 42 (2015) 409–423
http://dx.doi.org/10.1016/j.pop.2015.05.012
0095-4543/15/$ – see front matter © 2015 Elsevier Inc. All rights reserved.

primarycare.theclinics.com

necessary to wear very thick, heavy glasses. These glasses were inconvenient, unsightly, and induced a lot of prism caused by the thickness of the glass lenses. In 1949 a British ophthalmologist by the name of Harold Ridley noticed that plastic fragments from the cockpit canopies of fighter jets were well tolerated in the anterior chambers of the pilots who had been shot down. The idea was born of replacing the lens with a plastic one after the cataract was removed. In the decades since Dr Ridley's idea, IOLs have evolved in design, style, and material. Most modern IOLs are made of either acrylic or silicone. Current IOLs come in a spectrum of diopter powers. The biggest advantage to cataract surgery is that, in addition to restoring clarity to the eye by removing the cataract, the IOL placed can be optimized to correct much of a patient's refractive error. Thus, even patients who were strongly nearsighted or farsighted before cataract surgery will often have no to minimal correction required after, as the IOL is now correcting that error. The determination of IOL power is made by taking various measurements of the eye, specifically the axial length (the distance from the front of the cornea to fovea) and the curvature of the cornea, and then using regression formulas to calculate a power. Newer formulas also use anterior chamber depth, lens thickness, and corneal diameter to provide even more accurate results and, thus, a better chance of achieving emmetropia.

Prevalence and Epidemiology

Approximately 90% of blindness in developed countries can be attributed to cataracts. Prevalence of cataracts varies by age, race, and sex. In the United States, among the nursing home population, cataracts are a leading cause of low vision (as defined by visual acuity worse than 20/40 in the better-seeing eye), responsible for 37% of low vision among Caucasians and 54% of low vision among African Americans.[2] Among Americans, a visually significant cataract (visual acuity <20/40) is present in approximately 2.5% of those aged 40 to 49 years, 6.8% of those aged 50 to 59 years, 20.0% of those aged 60 to 69 years, 42.8% of those aged 70 to 79 years, and 68.3% of those aged greater than 80 years. The 3 subtypes of age-related cataracts (nuclear, cortical, and posterior subcapsular [PSC]) vary across populations. The term *nuclear cataract* describes the normal yellowing and sclerosis of the lens nucleus associated with aging. Cortical cataracts are wedge-shaped or spokelike opacities in the outer cortical layers of the lens. PSCs are plaquelike opacities along the posterior cortical layers. In the United States, nuclear cataracts are seen more commonly in Caucasians, whereas cortical cataracts are seen more commonly in African Americans; however, PSC cataracts are prevalent at roughly the same rate in both groups. Age-related cataracts may be further classified by the Lens Opacities Classification System III (LOCS III). This system, used at the slit lamp, grades the type and density of cataracts by comparing them with standard photographic color plates. Although LOCS III is a very accurate and reproducible way to grade the severity of cataracts, it is primarily used for research purposes to evaluate progression.[3] Cataracts affect nearly 22 million Americans aged 40 years and older. By 80 years of age, more than half of all Americans have cataracts. Direct medical costs for cataract treatment are estimated at $6.8 billion annually.[4] The prevalence of cataracts has a strong positive relationship with age.

ANATOMY AND PATHOLOGY

The lens is a transparent biconvex disk that sits behind the iris inside the eye (**Fig. 1**). The functions of the lens are to

1. Maintain its own clarity
2. Focus light
3. Provide accommodation

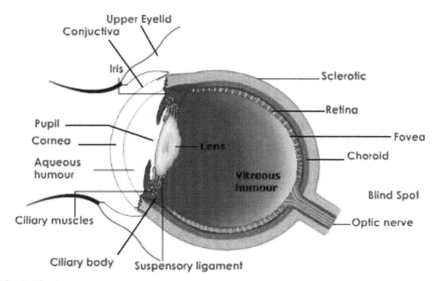

Fig. 1. The human eye.

It is suspended like a trampoline and is attached to the ciliary body, with fibers known as the zonules of Zinn. The developed lens is an avascular structure and is without innervation. Its metabolic needs are met by the adjacent aqueous humor. Histologically, the lens is composed of a single-layer, anterior, cuboidal, inverted epithelium that secretes an overlying thick basement membrane called the lens capsule to which the zonules attach. New cells are formed constantly during life and are laid down externally to the older cells. These newly formed cells differentiate into lens fibers. In doing so they stretch, lose their organelles, and dramatically increase the mass of cellular proteins. It is these changes that impart transparency to the lens. Because the epithelial cells are unable to shed and are instead differentiated into lens fibers, they are compacted centrally, with the oldest being in the center, or nucleus, of the lens. Without organelles these central cells are more susceptible to the photooxidative effects of aging. It is the photooxidative insults to these cells that lead to the discoloration and opacities in the lens known as a cataract. A cataract causes light to scatter when it passes through the lens, which decreases the amount of light to the retina.[5,6]

Types of Cataracts

There are several types of acquired cataracts: age related, secondary, and trauma related. Age related can be classified as nuclear, cortical, or PSC (**Fig. 2**). Secondary cataracts develop as a result of systemic disease or an ocular disease. Congenital cataracts can be genetic or disease related.

Age-related cataracts

- Nuclear: This type of cataract is the most common; it begins with a gradual hardening, yellowing, and sclerosis of the nucleus, which expands to other layers of the lens. This change is a normal aging change, though many factors are known to accelerate its formation.
- Cortical: This type tends to occur more often in persons with diabetes. It begins in the peripheral lens in the outer cortical layers and then slowly moves inward in a spoking pattern.

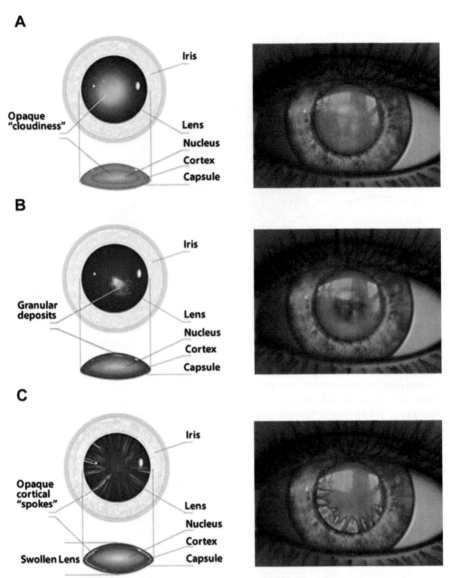

Fig. 2. Types of cataracts. (A) Nuclear cataract. (B) PSC cataract. (C) Cortical cataract.

- PSC: This type of cataract is plaquelike opacity of the back of the lens and can develop rapidly. Significant symptoms may not occur until the cataract is well developed. These cataracts are commonly associated with corticosteroid use.

Secondary cataracts

Several systemic or ocular diseases can predispose individuals to cataracts. Patients with diabetes have a high prevalence of cataracts.[5–7] Cataracts are among the earliest complications of diabetes mellitus. Klein and colleagues[8] demonstrated that patients with diabetes mellitus are 2 to 5 times more likely to develop cataracts than their nondiabetic counterparts; this risk may reach 15 to 25 times in diabetic patients who are less than 40 years of age.[9] Myotonic dystrophy, atopic dermatitis, neurofibromatosis, hypoparathyroidism, and Down syndrome, among many others, are also associated with cataract formation.

A variety of ocular conditions are also commonly associated with cataracts (**Fig. 3**). Uveitis, an inflammation of the inner eye, is commonly associated with cataracts. These cataracts may be caused both by inflammation and/or the steroids used to treat it.[10] Other ocular syndromes commonly associated with cataracts include acute congestive angle closure, high (pathologic) myopia, and hereditary fundus dystrophies, such as retinitis pigmentosa, Leber congenital amaurosis, gyrate atrophy, and Stickler syndrome.

Congenital
There are a variety of diseases and conditions linked to congenital cataracts. Diseases linked to cataract development include rubella, cytomegalovirus, varicella, syphilis, and toxoplasmosis. Genetic causes include autosomal-dominant congenital cataract, Lowe syndrome, and galactosemia.

Trauma
Both blunt and penetrating trauma are common causes of cataracts. Other types of trauma include electric shock, infrared radiation (eg, occupational exposure), and ionizing radiation (eg, for ocular tumors). These types can develop immediately following the traumatic event or insidiously over time. Because of the potential for injury to the zonules and other parts of the eye with blunt trauma, surgical repair of these cataracts can be more difficult and complications are more common.[11] Obtaining a detailed history of the type and extent of trauma is imperative for surgical planning.

SYMPTOMS

Cataracts most often present slowly and painlessly. Because of the insidious nature of progression many patients are often unaware of, and will not complain of, any dramatic changes in their vision. However, when asked about specific symptoms they will readily admit to difficulty. Thus, when completing a review of systems and questioning patients about their vision, it is important to ask specific closed questions instead of simply asking, how is your vision? Questions specifically designed to gauge the effect on activities of daily living and, thus, determine whether ophthalmic consultation is indicated include the following: Do you see well enough to safely drive at night? Are you able to easily read the print on your medication bottles?

The types of cataracts mentioned previously vary in how they present because of the different ways in which the opacities effect light transmission through the lens.

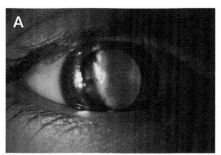 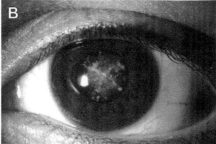

Fig. 3. Cataracts caused by various conditions. (A) Advanced diabetic cortical cataract. (B) Radiation cataract.

Nuclear sclerotic cataracts, with their yellowing and hardening of the central lens and resulting myopic shift, often present with diminished distance vision but few problems with near acuity. Patients may complain about difficulty seeing road signs or following a golf ball but have no problem reading a newspaper. Cortical cataracts, caused by the spoking of the peripheral lens, are more problematic in low light when the pupil naturally dilates to let more light in and involves the peripheral opacified lens in focusing light. This cataract commonly results in complaints of glare, especially when driving at night. PSC cataracts, caused by the opacity being central, are most bothersome in bright light or when the pupil is constricted, such as when reading because all focused light passes through the small pupillary opening and then the opacity immediately behind it. Symptoms tend to improve in low light when the pupil then dilates and light is able to pass around the cataract. Although this is a good rule of thumb, any visual complaint can be found with any type of cataract (**Fig. 4**).[12]

The most common complaints consistent with a worsening cataract are as follows:

- Blurred vision and/or glare, especially when driving at night
- Reduced visual acuity, contrast sensitivity, or color appreciation
- Increasing nearsightedness
- Monocular double vision or ghosting: seeing multiple images of one object

HISTORY

A thorough history is important when you have a patient who presents with symptoms of a cataract. The primary care physician's priority is to establish both the clinical suspicion for a cataract in light of a vision complaint and to determine a patient's suitability

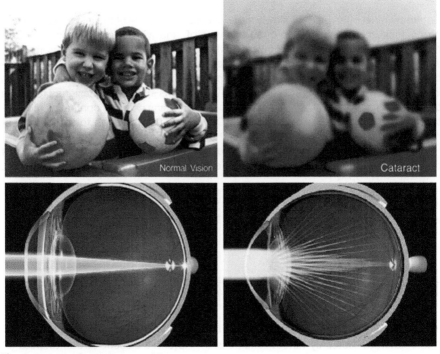

Fig. 4. Impact of cataracts on vision.

for surgery. Relevant aspects of a past medical history include previous eye conditions, previous ocular injuries or surgeries, concurrent ocular diseases, and genetic predispositions.

A history of medication use, specifically alpha-blocker use, such as tamsulosin hydrochloride (Flomax), is of critical importance for the primary care physician to pass onto the ophthalmologist as many patients do not know the medications they take. This class of medications can be very problematic during cataract surgery as they can cause intraoperative floppy iris syndrome (IFIS). This syndrome leads to a loss of tone of the iris causing progressive pupillary constriction during surgery resulting in iris trauma and inadequate visualization. As a result, complication rates are significantly higher in patients with IFIS. Unfortunately, stopping these medications before surgery does not necessarily lessen the chance of IFIS because of the permanent structural changes to the iris. However, the surgical technique can be adjusted to account for these changes as long as the ophthalmologist knows to expect them.[13]

Other conditions, such as obesity, alcohol consumption, smoking, hypertension, and known inflammatory markers, can all have an impact on the safety of and recovery from cataract surgery. The more relevant a history the primary care physician obtains, the more these factors can be taken into account to individualize a surgical plan and optimize the outcome.

WORKUP AND EVALUATION

In evaluating patients with visual complaints, the first step in evaluation by the primary care physician is the determination of visual acuity at both distance and near. Vision should be checked with the most current or best pair of glasses, and patients should be pushed to read the smallest line possible on the Snellen chart and near card. It should be noted that 20/20 or near-perfect vision does not preclude the presence of a cataract. Types of cataracts, specifically cortical, can present with a significant reduction in functional vision in glare situations (such as night driving); visual acuity testing alone will not reveal the full degree of visual disability.

If the primary physician is comfortable with a direct ophthalmoscope, it can be a very useful tool in both diagnosing a cataract and discerning other causes of the visual complaint. Depending on the comfort level of the primary physician, dilating the pupils (as long as no known history of narrow angles exists) with 2.5% phenylephrine and 1.0% tropicamide can greatly enhance the view of the lens. With the lens power set to zero, hold the ophthalmoscope approximately 12 inches from the eye. The reflection of light off of the retina will produce a bright red reflex. This reflex should be uniform in color and brightness. Any cataract change in the lens will show up as a dark spot against the red reflex.[12] Specifically, PSC and cortical cataracts are most readily discernable by this method (**Figs. 5** and **6**). Next, the ophthalmoscope should be used to evaluate the optic nerve and fundus, much easier if the pupils are dilated, for any retinal conditions that could also explain the vision complaints. The presence of any drusen, scarring, or hemorrhages should be noted.

A thorough eye examination by the primary care physician should include the following:

- Distance and near visual acuity with by Snellen letter, Tumbling E, or picture charts WITH newest or best glasses
- The external eyes for trauma or deformity
- Extraocular muscle movements
- The presence of an afferent papillary defect

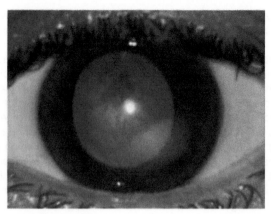

Fig. 5. PSC cataract retroillumination.

- Red reflex bilaterally
- Optic nerve and disk with the ophthalmoscope
- Ability to fixate on and follow or reach for moving object in preverbal patients

If the suspicion of a cataract exists, based on history, demographics, and/or examination findings a referral to ophthalmology should be made for further evaluation and management.

The lens is best examined with a dilated pupil by an ophthalmologist. **Table 1** includes diagnostic methods used by the ophthalmologist to evaluate cataracts.

MANAGEMENT AND TREATMENT
Nonsurgical Management of the Cataract

Although cataracts are ultimately a surgical condition, there are several nonsurgical treatment options that may be temporarily effective in optimizing visual function. First,

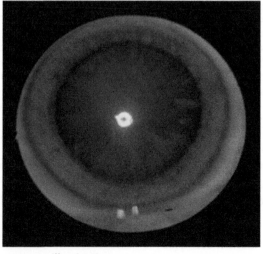

Fig. 6. Cortical cataract retroillumination.

Table 1 Ophthalmologic diagnostic modalities	
Slit lamp	A biomicroscope, used to visually examine the eye; used to detect the type and severity of cataract opacity within lens
Potential acuity meter or laser interferometer	Used to assess potential visual acuity with removal of cataract if other forms of ocular pathology exist
B-scan ultrasound	Used to detect retinal detachment or tumors if a cataract is so dense that it prevents retinal examination
Glare testing and contrast sensitivity testing	Used to quantitatively assess functional impact of glare or loss of contrast in cataracts

vision can often by improved with a careful refraction and a new pair of glasses for distance and near vision. For specific complaints of difficulty reading, increasing ambient lighting or increasing the power of the bifocal portion of the glasses can help. Although research is ongoing, there is currently no medical treatment to definitively treat or reverse cataract formation.

Surgical Management of Cataracts

The primary indication for cataract surgery is the patients' desire for improved visual function and the likelihood that cataract surgery will help them achieve that goal. The decision to proceed is not based on a specific level of acuity but on when patients and the physician determine that the diminished acuity from the cataracts interferes with daily activities.

Indications for Surgery

- Improve vision and overall functionality
- Address medical indications (eg, phacomorphic glaucoma)
- Facilitate management of fundus disease (eg, diabetic retinopathy) when posterior view is too poor to adequately diagnose and follow

Cost-effectiveness of Cataract Surgery

In the United States, each year, almost 1.5 million people have cataract surgery at a total estimated cost of $3.4 billion. However, the cost of not treating a cataract is much greater because of the effects of cataract-related vision loss on the ability to work and to function independently. Therefore, the optimal management of a cataract that is symptomatic and limiting to functionality is surgical removal.

Despite the large amount of money spent annually on cataract surgery, the quality-of-life gain is tremendous. One evaluation showed that monocular cataract surgery conferred a gain of 1.62 quality-adjusted life-years (QALYs), whereas bilateral cataract surgery conferred more than 2.8 QALYs of benefit.[5] Another student demonstrated that initial cataract surgery yielded an extraordinary 4567% financial return on investment to society over the 13-year model. This finding is even more reassuring given other data that cataract surgery is 34.4% less expensive than in 2000 and 85.0% less expensive than in 1985. However, for most ocular interventions, patient value gain occurs primarily because of improvement in quality of life. Cataract surgery in the first eye confers a 20.8% quality-of-life gain, more than double the 6.3% to 9.1% patient value gain in quality of life and length of life conferred by b-adrenergic blockers for the treatment of systemic arterial hypertension.[7]

Preoperative Assessment

A Cochrane review showed that routine preoperative testing does not increase the safety of cataract surgery. The analysis included 3 studies with a sufficient sample size and statistical power to investigate this claim. Reviews of the literature and practice guidelines found that commonly performed preoperative laboratory tests in adults preparing for elective surgeries have generally low predictive value. Before the conduct of this review, surveys of ophthalmologists in the United States and Canada in 1992 indicated that among ophthalmologists, ordering preoperative screening tests was common and that these tests were often ordered despite a lack of belief in their clinical value. Tests were sometimes ordered in the belief that other physicians required the test results or based on medicolegal concerns.

This review reported results for 21,531 total cataract surgeries. Among those, there were 707 total medical adverse events associated with cataract surgeries, including 61 hospitalizations and 3 deaths. Of the 707 medical adverse events reported, 353 occurred in the pretesting group and 354 occurred in the no-testing group. Most events were cardiovascular and occurred during the intraoperative period. Preoperative medical testing did not reduce the rate of intraoperative (odds ratio [OR] 1.02, 95% confidence interval [CI] 0.85–1.22) or postoperative medical adverse events (OR 0.96, 95% CI 0.74–1.24) compared with selective or no testing. Alternatives to routine preoperative medical testing have been proposed, including self-administered health questionnaires. Such avenues may lead to cost-effective means of identifying those at an increased risk of medical adverse events caused by cataract surgery. However, despite the rare occurrence, adverse medical events precipitated by cataract surgery remain a concern because of the multiple medical comorbidities among the age demographic of cataract surgery patients. The studies summarized in this review should assist recommendations for the standard of care of cataract surgery, at least in developed settings.

Currently, the Centers for Medicare and Medicaid Services, which covers most cataract surgeries in the United States, covers preoperative services that assess a beneficiary's fitness for surgery.[14] Although such services are covered, the American Academy of Ophthalmology's practice guidelines recommend testing on indication rather than routine preoperative medical testing.[15] In the United Kingdom, the Royal College of Ophthalmologists' guidelines[16] and National Health Service do not recommend routine preoperative medical testing (ie, blood tests and electrocardiograms) before cataract surgery. Similarly, the American Heart Association recommends against routine testing in patients undergoing low-risk procedures, such as cataract surgery.[17] Thus, although cataract surgery carries very low risks and routine testing is not recommended, preoperative medical evaluation by the primary care physician to determine overall fitness for the procedure is commonly sought based on known comorbidities. Contraindications to surgery include uncontrolled hypertension, hyperglycemia, unstable heart disease, systemic infections, or any respiratory issues. Patients with a variety of complex medical conditions can have cataract surgery performed as long as those conditions are stable. The primary care physician will often be asked to consult with the ophthalmologist and anesthesiologist before surgery if there are any concerns.

In general, patients taking aspirin or other anticoagulant drugs do not need to change their regimen before undergoing cataract extraction as there is generally no bleeding and minimal risk of any. Despite this, measures of control, such as the international normalized ratio, should be within the therapeutic range. However, retrobulbar and peribulbar anesthesia should be avoided in patients on anticoagulants. The surgeon should also be aware of other drugs patients may be taking, specifically tamsulosin hydrochloride (Flomax) and other alpha-1 antagonists.

Cataract Surgery

Before the surgery
Before cataract surgery, patients undergo a comprehensive ophthalmologic examination, including measurement of refraction, measurement of intraocular pressure, slit lamp examination, and examination of the retinal fundus with the pupils dilated. Other causes of impaired vision must be ruled out or taken into account, such as glaucoma, age-related macular degeneration, diabetic retinopathy, or optic nerve pathology. Glare effect can be measured by determining visual acuity under conditions of increased ambient lighting, which can greatly exacerbate cataract symptoms. In patients with coexisting eye problems, such as age-related macular degeneration, special testing and clinical judgment are needed to assess the potential value of cataract surgery.

Anesthesia for cataract surgery
Nearly all cataract operations in the United States are performed with light sedation along with a topical anesthesia. This technique is currently the most time-efficient and cost-efficient method. Retrobulbar and peribulbar injections have become less common because of a longer visual recovery and a higher risk of serious complications. Also, topical anesthesia does not affect vision and does not cause akinesia (temporary paralysis) of the eye, so many patients have useful and improved vision almost immediately after surgery. Some ophthalmologists are even eliminating intravenous sedation and are just using a small amount of oral sedation along with topical anesthesia. General anesthesia may be appropriate in patients who cannot cooperate because of advanced age, poor mental status, or severe claustrophobia. It is the extensive history provided by the primary care physician that is instrumental in determining the optimum anesthesia technique for each case.

Current surgical techniques
The 3 main techniques for cataract extraction today are intracapsular extraction, extracapsular extraction, and phacoemulsification. More than 99% of cataract surgeries in the United States are done with phacoemulsification.

Intracapsular cataract extraction
Intracapsular cataract extraction is the removal of the entire lens including the capsule, after which patients must wear special (ie, aphakic) eyeglasses because no IOL is implanted. This procedure is no longer used in developed countries except in rare cases, such as a partly dislocated lens. It has a high rate of intraoperative and postoperative complications, and the need for thick glasses or contacts makes it much less desirable.

Extracapsular cataract extraction
Extracapsular cataract extraction involves removing the opacified lens as a whole but leaving the capsule of the lens and its zonular attachments intact. The capsular bag then provides a scaffold for implantation of a synthetic lens. Although this method does allow implantation of an IOL, it requires a large incision at the corneal-scleral junction requiring sutures for closure and a longer recovery. Complication rates are also much higher than with phacoemulsification. This procedure is used for very mature cataracts that are too dense for phacoemulsification.

Phacoemulsification

Phacoemulsification is currently the most commonly used procedure for cataract extraction in the United States. This procedure is a less invasive version of extracapsular cataract extraction, developed by Charles Kelman in 1967, in which the lens nucleus is emulsified within its capsule using an ultrasonic probe inserted through a small (1.8–3.0 mm) incision. When constructed properly, the small wound size is self-sealing and precludes the need for a suture to close it. The advantages of phacoemulsification compared with regular extracapsular extraction are that the incision is smaller; the rates of intraoperative complications, such as vitreous loss and iris prolapse, are lower; the procedure time is shorter; and the time to visual recovery is faster. As with the other extracapsular approach, the capsular bag is maintained, allowing for easy placement of a synthetic lens implant (**Fig. 7**). Despite the rapid healing and rare complications of phacoemulsification, the eyes are generally operated on separately and done 1 to 4 weeks apart.

Postoperative Care

In uneventful phacoemulsification, the patients' vision will often return to normal within a few days. In order to speed visual recovery and prevent complications, patients are usually placed on a combination of drops after surgery. The most common regimen is an antibiotic, a steroid, and a nonsteroidal antiinflammatory drug. These medications are usually used for 3 to 6 weeks postoperatively. In addition, optimal recovery is achieved with a limitation of strenuous activity for a week or so. Activities such as weight lifting, heavy yard work, or impact sports are avoided. Because no sutures are placed, patients are also advised to avoid rubbing the eye and a plastic shield is often placed over the eye when sleeping to avoid inadvertent contact. If needed, a new glasses prescription can be given to patients in 1 to 3 weeks after both eyes are done.

Intraocular lenses

Once the cataract has been removed from the eye, there is the resulting loss of the focusing power (albeit blurry) that the cataractous lens provided. As a result, nearly

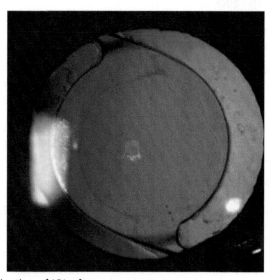

Fig. 7. Retroillumination of IOL after cataract surgery.

all modern cataract surgery involves the placement of an IOL during surgery, which replaces the natural lens and restores focusing power to the eye. These IOLs have evolved significantly since Dr Ridley first developed them. Some of the greatest advances in cataract surgery over the last decade have been in the types of IOLs that can be implanted (**Fig. 8**). Although a variety of IOL designs exist, they can be divided into three categories: monofocal, toric, and multifocal/pseudo-accomdative.[18] The types of IOLs are summarized in **Table 2**.

Because cataract surgery is only done one time, the determination of which type of IOL to implant is an important one. This decision is made by the surgeon and the patients together. Factors that play into this decision are the desired level of spectacle independence, amount of preexisting astigmatism, budget, and preexisting ocular comorbidities that may have an impact on final best-corrected vision after surgery.

PREVENTION

Prevention of cataracts primarily involves reducing risks. Significant research continues to be done on ways to slow the progression of cataracts. It is known that oxidative stress plays a large role on the cellular level in the formation cataracts. However, a large randomized study found that supplementation with vitamins C and E and beta-carotene had no impact on cataract formation.[19,20] Similar studies looking at aspirin, lutein, zeaxanthin, and glutathione found that they did not have any effect on slowing cataract formation either.[21] Although it is known that these antioxidant supplements have benefits to other systems, there are currently no data suggesting that their use should be predicated on a desire to prevent cataracts. However, research is ongoing.

More relevant to preventing cataracts is what exposures can be reduced. There is a well-established link between oral, topical, and ocular corticosteroid use and the development of PSC cataracts. The link between inhaled corticosteroids and PSC development is less certain.[22] Although cataracts are a correctable side effect of these medications, reducing the dose, duration, and strength can slow their development

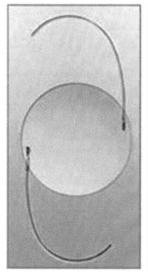 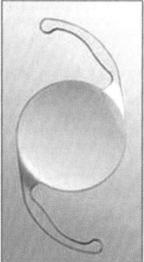 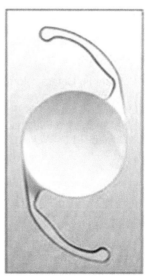

Fig. 8. Examples of IOLs.

Table 2 Types of IOLs	
Monofocal IOL	It is one focal length, usually targeting distance vision. Patients often still need reading glasses or bifocals for near activities. This type is the only type of IOL that insurance companies will reimburse for.
Toric IOL	It is astigmatism correcting. It can reduce/eliminate varying levels of preexisting corneal astigmatism reducing dependence on glasses or contacts after surgery for distance activities. It is not considered medically necessary and, therefore, not covered by insurance.
Multifocal and pseudoaccommodative IOLs	These IOLs are designed to minimize dependence of glasses after surgery at a variety of focal lengths by providing both distance and near vision. They do not correct astigmatism. They are not considered medically necessary and, therefore, not covered by insurance. They may have increased side effects, such as glare, haloes, and loss of contrast.

precluding the need for surgery, especially in younger patients. UV light has also been a well-established contributor to cataract development. There is evidence that reducing cumulative lifelong exposure to UV-B light can reduce cataract development, which is most easily achieved by wearing a hat and sunglasses with UV-B protection.[23] Smoking has been linked as a risk factor for the development of nuclear cataracts.[24] The Physicians' Health Study I showed, based on the first 5 years of follow-up, that current smokers of 20 or more cigarettes per day, compared with never smokers, had a 2-fold increased risk of cataract. Past smokers had a 15% increased risk of cataract development that was not found to be statistically significant.[25]

There are lifestyle factors that have been linked to decreased cataract formation. Increased physical activity, lower body mass index, and increased cardiorespiratory fitness have been found to have a preventative effect on cataract formation in men.[26] Among postmenopausal women, there is evidence that estrogen may play a protective role in reducing the incidence of age-related cataracts.[27]

REFERENCES

1. Shichi H. Cataract formation and prevention. Expert Opin Investig Drugs 2004; 13(6):691–701.
2. West SK, Munoz B, Schein OD, et al. Racial differences in lens opacities: the Salisbury Eye Evaluation (SEE) project. Am J Epidemiol 1998;148(11):1033–9.
3. Chylack LT Jr, Wolfe JK, Singer DM, et al. The lens opacities classification system III. The longitudinal study of cataract study group. Arch Ophthalmol 1993;111: 831–6.
4. Vision problems in the U.S.: prevalence of adult vision impairment and age-related eye disease in America. Prevent Blindness America and the National Eye Institute; 2008.
5. Yanoff M, Sassani J. Ocular pathology. London: Saunders; 2015. Print.
6. Kanski J, Bowling B. Synopsis of clinical ophthalmology. 3rd edition. St Louis (MO): Saunders; 2013.
7. Tsai JC. Oxford American handbook of ophthalmology. Oxford (UK): Oxford UP; 2011.

8. Klein BE, Klein R, Wang Q, et al. Older-onset diabetes and lens opacities. The Beaver Dam Eye Study. Ophthalmic Epidemiol 1995;2:49–55.
9. Bernth-Peterson P, Bach E. Epidemiologic aspects of cataract surgery. Frequencies of diabetes and glaucoma in a cataract population. Acta Ophthalmol 1983;61:406–16.
10. Hooper PL, Rao NA, Smith RE. Cataract extraction in uveitis patients. Surv Ophthalmol 1990;35(2):120–44.
11. Tasman W, Jaeger EA, editors. Traumatic cataract. In: Duane's clinical ophthalmology, vol. 1. Chicago: Lippincott Williams and Wilkins; 1997. p. 13–4.
12. American Academy of Ophthalmology. Basic and clinical science course: lens and cataract. 2004.
13. Chang DF, Osher RH, Wang L, et al. A prospective multicenter evaluation of cataract surgery in patients taking tamsulosin (Flomax). Ophthalmology 2007;114: 957–64.
14. Goldman HB, Kiffel S, Weinstock FJ. Cataract surgery and the primary care practitioner. Geriatrics 2009;64(5):19–22, 25–6.
15. American Academy of Ophthalmology. Routine pre-operative laboratory testing for patients scheduled for cataract surgery. 2000.
16. Au Eong KG. The Royal College of Ophthalmologists cataract surgery guidelines: what can patients see with their operated eye during cataract surgery? Eye 2002; 16(1):109–10.
17. Eagle KA, Berger PB, Calkins H, et al. ACC/AHA guideline update for perioperative cardiovascular evaluation for noncardiac surgery—executive summary: a report of the American College of Cardiology/American Heart Association task force on practice guidelines (committee to update the 1996 guidelines on perioperative cardiovascular evaluation for noncardiac surgery). J Am Coll Cardiol 2002;39(3):542–53 [Erratum appears in J Am Coll Cardiol 2006;47(11):2356].
18. Chayet A, Sandstedt C, Chang S, et al. Correction of myopia after cataract surgery with a light-adjustable lens. Ophthalmology 2009;116(8):1432–5.
19. Gritz DC, Srinivasan M, Smith SD. The antioxidants in prevention of cataracts study: effects of antioxidant supplements on cataract progression in South India. Br J Ophthalmol 2006;90:847–51.
20. West SK, Muñoz BE, Newland HS, et al. Lack of evidence for aspirin use and prevention of cataracts. Arch Ophthalmol 1987;105(9):1229–31.
21. Fernandez MM, Afshari NA. Nutrition and the prevention of cataracts. Curr Opin Ophthalmol 2008;19:66–70.
22. Jick SS, Vasilakis-Scaramozza C, Maier WC. The risk of cataract among users of inhaled steroids. Epidemiology 2001;12(2):229–34.
23. Meyer LM, Lofgren S, Holz FG, et al. Bilateral cataract induced by unilateral UVR-B exposure – evidence for an inflammatory response. Acta Ophthalmol 2013; 91(3):236–42.
24. Ye J, He J, Wang C, et al. Smoking and risk of age-related cataract: a meta-analysis. Invest Ophthalmol Vis Sci 2012;53(7):3885–95.
25. Christen WG, Glynn RJ, Ajani UA. Smoking cessation and risk of age-related cataract in men. JAMA 2000;284(6):713–6.
26. Zheng Selin J, Orsini N, Ejdervik Lindblad B, et al. Long-term physical activity and risk of age-related cataract: a population-based prospective study of male and female cohorts. Ophthalmology 2015;122(2):274–80.
27. Hales AM, Chamberlain CG, Murphy CR, et al. Estrogen protects lenses against cataract induced by transforming growth factor-beta (TGFbeta). J Exp Med 1997; 185(2):273–80.

Flashes and Floaters

Priya Sharma, MD[a], Jayanth Sridhar, MD[b], Sonia Mehta, MD[c],*

KEYWORDS

- Retinal tear • Retinal detachment • Migraine • Vitreous hemorrhage
- Posterior vitreous detachment

KEY POINTS

- Monocular flashes and floaters suggest an underlying ocular condition. In a middle-aged adult with no prior medical or ocular conditions, the most common cause is a posterior vitreous detachment. However, all patients deserve an immediate and thorough dilated examination with an ophthalmologist to evaluate for vitreous hemorrhage or a retinal tear.
- Bilateral flashes of specific size and pattern can reflect an underlying neurologic condition. Flashes preceding or following headache raise concern for migraine.
- New onset of floaters in a patient with known diabetic retinopathy or ischemic retinopathy raises concern for vitreous hemorrhage.
- Symptoms of pain or decreased vision in conjunction with flashes and floaters should be evaluated by an ophthalmologist immediately.

MONOCULAR SYMPTOMS

Monocular flashes and floaters often reflect an underlying ocular cause. The major monocular causes of flashes and floaters include vitreoretinal traction and vitreous hemorrhage. Additional, although less likely, ocular causes of flashes and floaters include uveitis, endophthalmitis, vitreous lymphoma, and retinal degenerations. Symptoms of pain or decreased vision in conjunction with flashes and floaters should be evaluated by an ophthalmologist immediately. Although rare, monocular flashes and floaters in conjunction with headache can reflect a subset of migraine referred to as retinal migraine. Retinal migraines are painless and temporary visual disturbances that present with auras, including scintillating scotoma, flashes, and other visual aberrations, but commonly occur unilaterally, unlike typical migraine. However,

Disclosures: The authors have no financial interest in the devices or medications in this document. The authors have no conflict of interest.
[a] Wills Eye Hospital, General Ophthalmology Service, 840 Walnut Street, Suite 800, Philadelphia, PA 19107, USA; [b] Mid Atlantic Retina, Retina Service, Wills Eye Hospital, 840 Walnut Street, Suite 1020, Philadelphia, PA 19107, USA; [c] Vitreoretinal Diseases & Surgery Service, Wills Eye Hospital, Department of Ophthalmology, Thomas Jefferson University Hospital, 840 Walnut Street, Suite 1020, Philadelphia, PA 19107, USA
* Corresponding author.
E-mail address: soniamehtamd@gmail.com

the focus of this article is the more common causes of monocular flashes and floaters in a primary care setting.

Vitreoretinal Traction

The vitreous is densely attached to the retina at the vitreous base, which is the area of 3 to 4 mm posterior to the ora serrata, at the junction of the retina and ciliary body. The vitreous is also attached, although less firmly, at the optic nerve, macula, and retinal vasculature. As the vitreous ages, it condenses and separates from the retina. As this separation happens, the vitreous can tug on the retina at these focal attachments. This retinal tugging causes photoreceptor and neuronal signals, leading to flashes. Floaters occur because of opacities in the vitreous media that cast shadows on the underlying retina. The most common cause of a floater in the setting of vitreoretinal traction is a posterior vitreous detachment, which reflects vitreous separation from the optic nerve head. The remnant of this attachment is called a Weiss ring (**Fig. 1**), or an opaque area in the posterior vitreous directly over the optic nerve that is circular in configuration and reflects the site of prior attachment. Floaters can also be a sign of hemorrhage, and can occur if the vitreous tugging is forceful or unsuccessful, thereby causing vasculature injury or a retinal tear.

Posterior vitreous detachment

Disease description Posterior vitreous detachment (PVD) is a common cause for monocular flashes and floaters in middle-aged adults. However, it is not limited to middle age, and can occur in all age groups, in association with high myopia, ocular trauma, or prior ocular surgery.

Definition PVD refers to the separation of the vitreous from the retina posterior to the vitreous base.

Prevalence/incidence The prevalence of PVD increases with age. It is generally rare in emmetropic patients less than 40 years of age, but by the age of 90 years, the reported prevalence ranges from 57% to 86%.[1,2]

Risk factors Risk factors for PVD include age, myopia (near-sightedness), prior ocular surgery, prior ocular laser therapy, ocular trauma, and inflammatory ocular disorders.

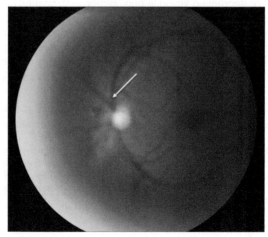

Fig. 1. Fundus photograph showing a Weiss ring (*arrow*) seen in a posterior vitreous detachment. The vitreous is in focus and therefore the background retinal blood vessels and optic nerve are purposely blurred.

Symptom criteria
There are several symptoms of PVD. Peripheral flashes that typically last for a few seconds are often noted. In addition, floaters are a common complaint, typically with a symptomatic opaque floater that is mobile in the patient's view (this reflects the presence of a Weiss ring). There is typically no central or peripheral loss of visual acuity.

Clinical findings
Physical examination Before referral, a brief ophthalmologic examination should be performed in any patient suspected of having a PVD. This brief examination should consist of visual acuity, pupillary reaction, and confrontation visual fields. After this, referral should be made immediately to an ophthalmologist, because comprehensive slit lamp and dilated fundus examinations are needed. Slit lamp examination is important, with special attention to the presence of so-called tobacco dust in the anterior vitreous and the presence of a Weiss ring (see **Fig. 1**; the white vitreous condensation reflects attachment of the vitreous to the peripapillary area). In addition, dilated fundus examination with indirect ophthalmoscopy and scleral depression of the affected eye in 360°[3] is critical to rule out any retinal tears or breaks.

Diagnostic modalities Diagnosis of PVD typically relies on slit lamp examination and indirect ophthalmoscopy with scleral depression to show successful detachment of the vitreous from the retina, without any other apparent ocular disorder. Scleral depression refers to the technique of indenting the anterior globe to be able to visualize it during indirect ophthalmoscopy.

Comorbidities PVD can be associated with a retinal tear or a retinal detachment.[3–5] Therefore, all patients should be evaluated by an ophthalmologist for concurrent retinal tear or retinal detachment.

Management goals
The most common complication of a PVD is a retinal tear, often a peripheral tear near the ora serrata. If a tear develops at this area, vitreous gel can get under the tear and lift the retina off the underlying epithelium, causing a retinal detachment. Therefore, the primary goal of managing a PVD is to rule out any underlying retinal tear or break.

Referral strategies
All patients should be referred to a general ophthalmologist or retinal specialist within 24 to 72 hours of onset of symptoms for a dilated fundus examination with scleral depression.

Self-management strategies
The patient should return for a repeat examination immediately if there are any increasing floaters, worsening flashes, or any loss of peripheral vision (commonly referred to as curtains or shades over vision). These symptoms are commonly referred to as retinal detachment warning signs.

Comanagement goals: evaluation, adjustment, recurrence
Most patients with PVD present with PVD in the fellow eye within 3 years.[6]

Summary
PVD is a common cause for monocular flashes and floaters in a middle-aged to elderly adult. It symptomatically presents as an opaque mobile spot (reflecting the Weiss ring in the vitreous gel) in the absence of any other ocular disorder. Care must be taken to rule out an underlying retinal tear or break.

Retinal tears and detachment

Disease description Retinal tears are defects in the retina that develop commonly from traction (**Fig. 2**). This traction can occur during a PVD, as described earlier. Tears from this mechanism are typically horseshoe in configuration, with a flap that reflects the retina that was tightly adherent to vitreous. As the flap enlarges, liquefied vitreous can travel underneath the flap and underneath the neurosensory retina, creating a large area of subretinal fluid that can expand and lead to a rhegmatogenous retinal detachment. There are other forms of retinal detachment (exudative and tractional), but the focus here is on the rhegmatogenous variant.

Definition A retinal tear is a small localized defect in the neurosensory retina, without an extensive amount of subretinal fluid.

A retinal detachment refers to the presence of an extensive amount of subretinal fluid elevating the retina above the underlying choroid.

Prevalence/incidence Nontraumatic retinal detachment has been reported to occur in approximately 1 in 10,000 people per year,[7,8] with an increased risk with myopia.[9]

Risk factors Risk factors for retinal tears and/or retinal detachments include high myopia, lattice degeneration, prior trauma, and PVD.[3,9,10]

Symptom criteria

Symptoms of retinal tears and/or retinal detachments include flashes, floaters, and loss of peripheral vision, which can be progressive and can help to localize the detachment. Loss of peripheral vision is often described as a shade or curtain that is obscuring the vision. Increasing amounts of subretinal fluid, and hence more elevation of the retina off of the underlying choroid, produce denser field defects. In addition, patients may complain of hazy vision caused by vitreous debris.

Clinical findings

Physical examination Similarly to a PVD, a brief ophthalmologic examination should be performed before referral in patients suspected of having a retinal tear or detachment. This brief examination should consist of visual acuity, pupillary reaction, and confrontation visual fields. Immediate referral should be made to an ophthalmologist

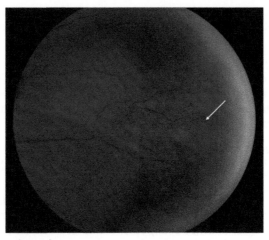

Fig. 2. A retinal tear (*arrow*).

for a full ophthalmologic examination, including slit lamp examination, with special attention to presence of tobacco dust (this represents liberated retinal pigment epithelial cells that have been released in the setting of a retinal tear) in the anterior vitreous and the presence of a Weiss ring. Dilated fundus examination with indirect ophthalmoscopy and scleral depression of the affected eye in 360° is crucial to locate the tear or detachment and define its characteristics.

Rating scales Rhegmatogenous retinal detachments (**Fig. 3**) are stratified into 2 main varieties. The first variety is macula-off, which describes a retinal detachment that extends to the macula and elevates it off of the retinal pigment epithelium, causing poor visual acuity. The second variety is macula-on, which describes a retinal detachment that does not involve the macula and can present with intact visual acuity.

Diagnostic modalities The major diagnostic modality consists of a slit lamp examination and indirect ophthalmoscopy with scleral depression, looking for characteristics of retinal tear and/or detachment.

Comorbidities In rare instances, retinal detachments can be associated with an underlying ocular malignancy (ie, exudative retinal detachment). All retinal detachments without a clear tear or with a suspicious clinical history or examination should have B-scan ultrasonography and/or referral to an ocular oncologist to evaluate for any underlying malignancy causing elevation of the retina.

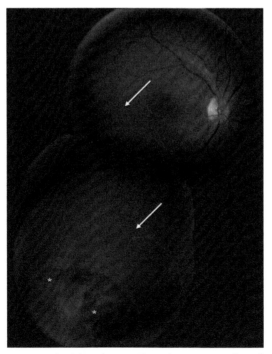

Fig. 3. A rhegmatogenous retinal detachment. Note the presence of a retinal break (*asterisks*) and fluid under the retina (*arrows*).

Management goals

If there is enough suspicion for a retinal detachment, the patient should be kept nothing by mouth and sent to a retinal specialist. Photoreceptor degeneration and vision loss can be minimized with early intervention, thus referral should not be delayed.[11]

Referral strategies

All suspected retinal detachments should be sent to an ophthalmologist or retinal specialist for evaluation within 24 hours.

Comanagement goals: evaluation, adjustment, recurrence

Patients with retinal detachments should have the fellow eye examined carefully, including a dilated examination with scleral depression, for any concurrent holes, tears, or detachments.

Summary

Retinal tears and/or detachments are among the most serious causes of monocular flashes and floaters. Care should be taken to get a thorough history and examination, and, if concerned, refer to a retinal specialist immediately.

Vitreous Hemorrhage

Introduction

Vitreous hemorrhage is another common cause of monocular floaters among patients presenting to a physician's office. Key findings in the patient's symptoms, past history, and clinical examination can help to diagnose vitreous hemorrhage, as well as clarify the cause of the vitreous hemorrhage.

Disease description Vitreous hemorrhage is painless loss of vision caused by blood products from normal or abnormal retinal vasculature. Vitreous hemorrhage can occur in isolation or secondary to many underlying ocular and systemic diseases.

Definition Vitreous hemorrhage refers to leakage of blood or blood products from a retinal vessel around and into the vitreous gel.

Prevalence/incidence Vitreous hemorrhage occurs in 7 in 100,000 cases.[12]

Risk factors There are many risk factors for vitreous hemorrhage, including retinal tear, PVD with retinal vascular tear, retinal detachment, diabetes, trauma, leukemia, macular degeneration, choroidal melanoma, sickle cell retinopathy, retinopathy of prematurity, prior vein or artery occlusion, and retinal artery macroaneurysm.

Symptom criteria

Vitreous hemorrhage typically presents as painless loss of vision in 1 eye. In the setting of trauma, neovascular glaucoma, or increased intraocular pressure, pain may be associated. Other symptoms include multiple visualized floaters (cobwebs) in vision, dark streaks or lines in vision, and/or cloudy vision or visual haze. If the vitreous hemorrhage is mild and localized, patient may complain of only a few spots in their vision. However, more extensive vitreous hemorrhage can cause almost complete loss of vision in the affected eye.

Clinical findings

Physical examination Before referral in a patient suspected of having a vitreous hemorrhage (**Fig. 4**), a brief ophthalmologic examination should be performed, consisting of visual acuity, pupillary reaction, and intraocular pressure calculation via handheld or

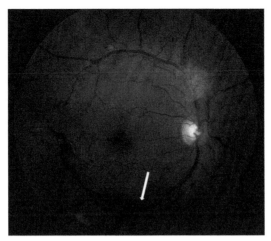

Fig. 4. A small inferior vitreous hemorrhage (*arrow*) from proliferative diabetic retinopathy.

portable tonometry. Immediate referral should be made to an ophthalmologist for slit lamp examination, dilated fundus examination with indirect ophthalmoscopy, and ocular ultrasonography.

Rating scales No consistent grading scale has been adopted, although grading of vitreous hemorrhage is often based on clock hours involved and presence or absence of a red reflex. A proposed grading scale is shown in **Fig. 5**.[13]

Diagnostic modalities Any patient with concurrent severe headache should be evaluated for Terson syndrome (concurrent subarachnoid hemorrhage with secondary extension of the bleeding into the ipsilateral vitreous cavity) with an emergent computed tomography scan and hospitalization if needed. Patients with dense vitreous hemorrhage that obscures the posterior pole and retina should have B-scan ultrasonography of the eye, which uses acoustic sound waves to recreate an image of the eye (**Fig. 6**). B-scan ultrasonography can help elucidate underlying causes of vitreous hemorrhage.

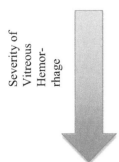

Severity of Vitreous Hemorrhage

Grade 1: 1 to 5 peripheral clock hours involved

Grade 2: 6 to 10 peripheral clock hours involved or involvement of the posterior equator

Grade 3: Presence red reflex

Grade 4: Dense vitreous hemorrhage without red reflex

Fig. 5. Grading scale for vitreous hemorrhage. (*Adapted from* Lieberman RM, Gow JA, Grill LR. Development and implementation of a vitreous hemorrhage grading scale. Retin Physician 2006. Available at: http://www.retinalphysician.com/articleviewer.aspx?articleID 5100200.)

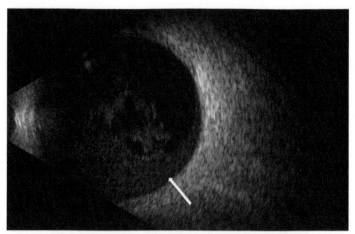

Fig. 6. B-scan ultrasonography of the eye showing acoustic hyperdensity in the vitreous (*arrow*), corresponding with vitreous hemorrhage. The retina appears flat. The cause of this vitreous hemorrhage was proliferative diabetic retinopathy.

Comorbidities Vitreous hemorrhage can be found in association with a PVD, retinal tear, or retinal detachment. Other systemic comorbidities that can be associated with vitreous hemorrhage include diabetes (see **Fig. 4**), blood disorders, hypertension, underlying inflammatory/autoimmune conditions, and in rare cases systemic leukemia.

Management goals

Care should be taken to determine the underlying cause for the vitreous hemorrhage. Often, this is not obvious immediately, and a retinal disorder can be obscured by the dense hemorrhage. In these cases, B-scan ultrasonography may be helpful.

Referral strategies

Referral should be made within 24 hours to an ophthalmologist or retinal specialist. Patients on Coumadin should have an International Normalized Ratio drawn, and patients with any concerning systemic history for leukemia should have a complete blood count.

Management strategies

All patients are advised to keep the head upright to allow the blood in the vitreous to pool inferiorly. Care should be taken not to bend or do any heavy lifting. Any blood thinners, including aspirin or nonsteroidal antiinflammatory drugs (NSAIDs), that are nonessential should be discontinued. Serial B-scan ultrasonography may be undertaken in patients who have a dense, slow-to-clear vitreous hemorrhage.

Summary

Vitreous hemorrhage presents as a spectrum, from floaters to a dense loss of vision. It can reflect a variety of underlying ocular or systemic conditions. After diagnosis, care should be taken to determine and treat the underlying cause of the hemorrhage.

BINOCULAR SYMPTOMS

Binocular flashes and floaters of a specific pattern generally reflect a neurologic cause. Binocular flashes and floaters most commonly suggest visual auras of migraine headache. These symptoms typically occur before or following a headache. Other causes of binocular flashes and floaters include occipital stroke, transient ischemic attack, syncope, hallucinations, and intracranial injury/hemorrhage.

Migraine Aura

Introduction
Disease description Migraine is a common and episodic headache disorder that is characterized by severe headache in addition to nausea and photosensitivity. It can be associated with an aura, or a sensory disturbance preceding headache, which occurs in approximately one-third of patients with migraine headaches.[14] Occasionally, aura occurs following headache or even in the absence of migraine.

Definition Migraine refers to a severe headache that occurs episodically in predisposed patients. The symptoms of migraine can be remembered with the evidence-based mnemonic POUND (**Box 1**).[15]

Aura refers to any sensory abnormality that occurs preceding or following a migraine. Duration is typically less than an hour and is completely reversible.

Risk factors Risk factors for migraine include family history, gender (women more than men), age (adolescents), and hormonal changes.

Symptom criteria
Typical migraine auras begin as a small area of visual loss or brightness that slowly expands over minutes to involve a quadrant of vision. Zigzagging colored lines can appear. The aura is often shimmering and travels throughout the visual field. Occasionally, patients experience loss of a hemifield of vision.

Clinical findings
Physical examination Physical examination should include pupillary examination, visual acuity, complete neurologic examination including cranial nerve examination, and direct ophthalmoscopy to evaluate nerve margins.

Management goals
Symptoms of new or worsening migraine headaches should be evaluated with brain MRI to evaluate for any underlying brain tumor, hemorrhage, or other nidus for headache, especially in the presence of any focal neurologic findings.[16]

Referral strategies
Referral should be made to a neurologist within 1 to 2 weeks for management. An examination by an ophthalmologist should also be performed within 1 to 2 weeks to evaluate for papilledema.

Box 1
POUND mnemonic for migraine symptoms
Pulsatile quality of headache
One-day duration (4–72 hours)
Unilateral location
Nausea or vomiting
Disabling intensity
From Wilson JF. In the clinic. Migraine. Ann Intern Med. 2007;147(9):ITC11-2; [Erratum appears in Ann Intern Med 2008;148(5):408].

Pharmacologic strategies

NSAIDs, aspirin, or other over-the-counter analgesics can be used in mild migraine headaches for symptomatic relief.[17] Avoid over-the-counter pain medications for prolonged treatment of migraine headaches. In addition, antiemetics may be used for symptomatic relief of nausea or vomiting. Treatment should also be initiated with triptans, ergotamines, or other long-term migraine-specific medications for management of underlying migraine headaches.

Nonpharmacologic strategies

Triggers of migraine should be identified, to help avoid future triggers.

Summary

Bilateral zigzag flashes of a specific pattern typically reflect an underlying neurologic cause, especially in conjunction with headache. For new-onset migraine with aura, or a patient with worsening headaches, MRI may be indicated.

REFERENCES

1. Akiba J. Prevalence of posterior vitreous detachment in high myopia. Ophthalmology 1993;100(9):1384–8.
2. Weber-Krause B, Eckardt C. Incidence of posterior vitreous detachment in the elderly. Ophthalmologe 1997;94(9):619–23 [in German].
3. D'Amico DJ. Clinical practice. Primary retinal detachment. N Engl J Med 2008; 359(22):2346–54.
4. Hikichi T, Trempe CL, Schepens CL. Posterior vitreous detachment as a risk factor for retinal detachment. Ophthalmology 1995;102(4):527–8.
5. Jaffe NS. Complications of acute posterior vitreous detachment. Arch Ophthalmol 1968;79(5):568–71.
6. Hikichi T, Yoshida A. Time course of development of posterior vitreous detachment in the fellow eye after development in the first eye. Ophthalmology 2004; 111(9):1705–7.
7. Wilkes SR, Beard CM, Kurland LT, et al. The incidence of retinal detachment in Rochester, Minnesota, 1970-1978. Am J Ophthalmol 1982;94(5): 670–3.
8. Haimann MH, Burton TC, Brown CK. Epidemiology of retinal detachment. Arch Ophthalmol 1982;100(2):289–92.
9. Risk factors for idiopathic rhegmatogenous retinal detachment. The Eye Disease Case-Control Study Group. Am J Epidemiol 1993;137(7):749–57.
10. Byer NE. Long-term natural history of lattice degeneration of the retina. Ophthalmology 1989;96(9):1396–401.
11. Sarrafizadeh R, Hassan TS, Ruby AJ, et al. Incidence of retinal detachment and visual outcome in eyes presenting with posterior vitreous separation and dense fundus-obscuring vitreous hemorrhage. Ophthalmology 2001;108(12): 2273–8.
12. Spraul CW, Grossniklaus HE. Vitreous hemorrhage. Surv Ophthalmol 1997;42(1): 3–39.
13. Lieberman RM, Gow JA, Grill LR. Development and implementation of a vitreous hemorrhage grading scale. Retin Physician 2006. Available at: http://www.retinalphysician.com/articleviewer.aspx?articleID=100200.
14. Lipton RB, Stewart WF, Diamond S, et al. Prevalence and burden of migraine in the United States: data from the American Migraine Study II. Headache 2001; 41(7):646–57.

15. Wilson JF. In the clinic. Migraine. Ann Intern Med 2007;147(9). ITC11-1–16; [Erratum appears in Ann Intern Med 2008;148(5):408].
16. Morey SS. Headache consortium releases guidelines for use of CT or MRI in migraine work-up. Am Fam Physician 2000;62(7):1699–701.
17. Gilmore B, Magdalena M. Treatment of acute migraine headache. Am Fam Physician 2011;83(3):271–80.

Glaucoma

Anand V. Mantravadi, MD[a],*, Neil Vadhar, MD[b]

KEYWORDS

- Glaucoma • Open angle • Angle closure • Screening • Diagnosis • Management
- Referral

KEY POINTS

- Glaucoma is the second leading cause of blindness both in the United States and worldwide and is the world's most common cause of irreversible blindness.
- The disease can be characterized into 2 major subtypes based on the status of the internal drainage system: open angle and angle closure.
- Risk factors for open-angle glaucoma include family history, increased intraocular pressure (IOP), older age (>60), increased cup-to-disc ratio, and thinner central corneas. Risk factors for angle-closure glaucoma include hyperopia (smaller eye), older age, female gender, and Asian ethnicity.
- Angle-closure glaucoma can present acutely with symptoms of pain or decreased vision and nausea or chronically without symptoms, similar to open-angle glaucoma.
- Glaucoma is a clinical diagnosis, based on characteristic optic nerve changes associated with corresponding visual field deficits, regardless of IOP.
- Management of glaucoma includes topical and oral medical therapies, laser modalities, and surgical management, all aimed at lowering IOP.

INTRODUCTION

Glaucoma is an optic neuropathy defined by characteristic optic disc damage and visual field loss for which IOP is a major modifiable risk factor. It is a significant global health problem and the second leading cause of blindness both in the United States and worldwide.[1,2] Worldwide, glaucoma affects 67 million people, 10% of whom are blind bilaterally.[1] In the United States, more than 2 million Americans are affected, with 120,000 blind as a result, costing approximately $1.5 billion in expenses.[2–4] Glaucoma is responsible for 11% of the cases of blindness and is the leading cause of blindness in African Americans.[5,6] With the aging population, the incidence and burden of glaucoma are expected to rise to even more significant levels.

No financial interest in material.
[a] Glaucoma Service, Wills Eye Hospital, 840 Walnut Street, Suite 1110, Philadelphia, PA 19107, USA; [b] Jefferson Medical College of Thomas Jefferson University, Philadelphia, PA, USA
* Corresponding author.
E-mail address: a_mantravadi@yahoo.com

Prim Care Clin Office Pract 42 (2015) 437–449
http://dx.doi.org/10.1016/j.pop.2015.05.008
0095-4543/15/$ – see front matter © 2015 Elsevier Inc. All rights reserved.

Glaucoma is often divided into 2 major subtypes, open angle and angle closure, both of which result in characteristic optic nerve degeneration. Both can be further subdivided into primary or secondary due to some other inciting factors. Secondary glaucoma can result from many other pathologic processes, including but not limited to vasculopathic, malignant, and traumatic.

Open-angle glaucoma is a chronic, insidious process. Patients are often unaware of their disease until vision loss has progressed significantly, known as the "sneak thief of sight." Early diagnosis remains a challenge given the insidious nature of the onset of this process and, therefore, formal ophthalmologic evaluation of any patient with risk factors is critical for prompt detection.

In contrast, angle-closure glaucoma can be an acute process with more immediate signs and symptoms but may also present insidiously and tends to be a more visually destructive subtype. It accounts for approximately half the cases of glaucoma worldwide and, when acute, is considered an ocular emergency because loss of vision can occur within hours to days.[7] By 2020, it is estimated that there will be 21 million cases of primary angle-closure glaucoma, with 5.3 million blind bilaterally.[8]

PATHOPHYSIOLOGY OF GLAUCOMA

The optic nerve is the site of degenerative damage in glaucoma (**Figs. 1** and **2**). The characteristic appearance of glaucomatous optic neuropathy is described as cupping or acquired focal or general loss of neural retinal rim tissue. Various systems to clinically denote the degree of optic nerve damage due to glaucoma have been described, including cup-to-disc ratio and disc damage likelihood scales. The precise inciting mechanism for the cascade of cellular damage resulting in glaucomatous optic neuropathy is not clear and is likely a complex interplay of several factors, including structural susceptibility and vascular. Elevated IOP is an important risk factor for developing glaucomatous optic neuropathy, and, furthermore, the rate at which glaucoma damage progresses is higher at greater levels of IOP.[9,10]

Normally, the IOP is a balance of aqueous humor production by the ciliary body and aqueous humor drainage through the internal outflow system. A major component of the outflow system is the trabecular meshwork located in an area denoted as the

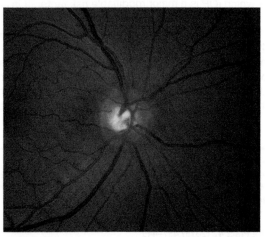

Fig. 1. Healthy optic nerve right eye. (*Courtesy of* Wills Eye Hospital Diagnostic Center, Philadelphia, PA; with permission.)

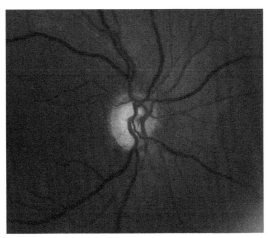

Fig. 2. Glaucomatous disc right eye with asymmetric neuroretinal rim inferiorly. (*Courtesy of* Wills Eye Hospital Diagnostic Center, Philadelphia, PA; with permission.)

angle. In open-angle glaucoma, the major site of resistance to outflow of aqueous humor is thought to be at the level of the trabecular meshwork. The consequence of outflow dysfunction is, therefore, elevated IOPs. Several robust randomized controlled clinical trials have clearly demonstrated the value in IOP lowering by a variety of methods in reducing the rate of glaucoma damage and consequential visual field loss.[9–12] Despite this evidence, it is clear that there is a certain individual susceptibility to developing optic nerve damage.[13] Above-average IOP may in some cases never lead to glaucoma damage. In others, if there is an inherent high susceptibility of the optic nerve to damage, glaucomatous optic neuropathy can develop even without elevation in IOPs—a common entity described as normal tension glaucoma.[14] Thus, although all current treatments are aimed at lowering IOP as a modifiable risk factor, it is not a part of the definition of glaucoma.

In contrast, in angle-closure glaucoma, the trabecular meshwork is physically obstructed typically by the iris (**Fig. 3**).[15,16] This is a result of a complex pathologic

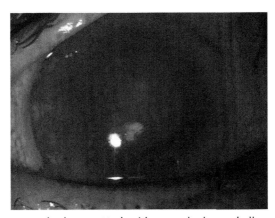

Fig. 3. Eye with acute angle-closure attack with corneal edema, shallow anterior chamber, and mid-dilated pupil. (*Courtesy of* Wills Eye Glaucoma Service, Philadelphia, PA; with permission.)

interaction of several intraocular structures and commonly can occur in smaller anatomic eyes.[17] Sudden obstruction leads to rapid rises in IOP and profound acute visual loss and discomfort, requiring urgent evaluation and treatment.

Risk Factors

For the development of open-angle glaucoma, many risk factors have been implicated (**Box 1**). The clearly established risk factors include increased IOP, older age, increased cup-to-disc ratio, and thinner central corneas.[9] The African American population in this country is a high-risk group with up to 6 times the incidence compared with white ancestry.[18] First-degree family history of glaucoma has been found to increase risk by 2.2 to 3.7 fold.[19]

In angle-closure glaucoma, risk factors include older age, female gender, and Asian ethnicity (**Box 2**).[20–22] Additionally, hyperopic (far-sighted) patients are at an increased risk for angle-closure glaucoma due to smaller depth and volume of the eye.[17] Those at risk for angle-closure glaucoma with crowded angle structures can develop an attack precipitated by pupillary dilation either spontaneously or pharmacologically.[23] Therefore, many systemic medications with glaucoma warnings are referring typically to the potential for pupillary dilation as a side effect, which may induce an acute attack in those at risk for developing angle-closure glaucoma (**Box 3**).

Clinical Signs and Symptoms of Glaucoma

Because of the chronic nature of open-angle glaucoma, patients typically present with slow, progressive, irreversible, painless loss of peripheral vision. Because of its insidious nature, more than 50% of patients are unaware of their condition.[1,3] Typically, patients with glaucoma may present with characteristic optic nerve changes and corresponding visual field loss. The IOPs may or may not be elevated.

Patients suffering from angle-closure glaucoma acutely present with symptoms. The affected eye typically is red or hyperemic, teary, and painful, with sudden blurring of vision. Patients may complain of halos around lights secondary to corneal edema from an acute rise in IOP. The elevated IOP may cause headache, nausea, and vomiting as well. On examination, patients present with a shallow anterior chamber and a fixed, mid-dilated pupil. The pupil may also be asymmetrically shaped, be poorly reactive, and have an afferent defect that is a reflection of optic nerve dysfunction.[24]

DIAGNOSIS

The diagnosis of glaucoma is typically made by clinical evaluation, including slit lamp biomicroscopy, measurement of IOP, careful assessment of the anterior chamber angle and the optic nerve, and functional visual field testing (**Fig. 4**).[25] Structural

---

Box 1
Risk factors for primary open-angle glaucoma

Elevated IOP

Older age

Increased cup-to-disc ratio

Thinner central cornea

African American race

Family history

Box 2
Risk factors for angle-closure glaucoma
Older age
Female gender
Asian ethnicity
Hyperopia

testing that quantifies various aspects of the optic nerve architecture compared with age-matched normal group is helpful. Clinically evident characteristic optic nerve damage and associated visual field deficits clearly establish the diagnosis. Optic nerve damage can occur, however, without visual field loss in the early to moderate stages; therefore, careful documentation of the appearance of the optic nerve should be made. The primary method for monitoring disease development or progression is through the use of photography and other optic nerve imaging modalities.[25] In the primary care setting, direct ophthalmoscopy may be used to assess the optic nerve; however, it alone is not sufficient to make the diagnosis.[26]

Progressive neuroretinal rim loss of the optic nerve, resulting in characteristic cupping is the structural hallmark of glaucoma. Features suggestive of glaucoma include enlargement of the central cup, focal thinning or notching of the neural rim, or hemorrhages of the optic nerve.[25,27]

Distinguishing between open-angle and angle-closure glaucoma hinges on careful optical assessment of the anterior chamber angle using a prism lens called gonioscopy (**Fig. 5**). In skilled hands, this represents the gold standard of angle evaluation to identify those at risk for angle-closure glaucoma.[24] The interexaminer reproducibility and sensitivity of gonioscopy to examine the angle has been established. Modalities using ultrasound and light (optical coherence tomography) to image the structures within the angle can be supporting and hold promise for screening as image quality improves (**Fig. 6**).[28]

Screening and Prevention

Thus far, the value of a screening program and sound guidelines have yet to be established because of the challenges in proper diagnosis and the lack of a singular test to

Box 3
Potential angle closure–inducing medications
α/β-Adrenergic agonists
Anticholinergics
Antihistamines
Cholinergic agents
Tricyclic antidepressants
Selective serotonin reuptake inhibitors
Serotonin norepinephrine reuptake inhibitors
Data from Lai JS, Gangwani RA. Medication induced acute angle-closure attack. Hong Kong Med J 2012;18:139.

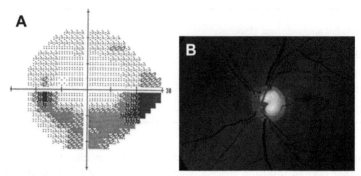

Fig. 4. Visual field left eye: perimetry is a standard tool to identify thresholds of light sensitivity compared with age-matched normal. In glaucoma, common patterns of visual field loss are arc-shaped patterns of visual field loss that corresponding to neuroretinal rim loss of optic nerve, which typically respect the horizontal meridians. In contrast, certain disorders, such as stroke, that may affect the visual pathways may respect the horizontal meridian and be homonymous. In this figure, the visual field (*A*) demonstrates an inferior arcuate scotoma that corresponds to the structural findings of glaucomatous superior optic nerve rim degeneration/loss (*B*). (*Courtesy of* Wills Eye Hospital Diagnostic Center, Philadelphia, PA; with permission.)

capture disease adequately. Targeting high-risk populations and first-degree relatives of those with disease can be important for early diagnosis and management to prevent disease progression.[25] IOP, as discussed previously, although important to the development of disease and rate of disease progression, is not by any means diagnostic of glaucoma. People can certainly have above average IOPs without developing glaucoma and in contrast, people with average IOPs can develop glaucoma.[13]

Currently, the American Academy of Ophthalmology recommends a complete eye examination for patients greater than or equal to 40 years of age or older (**Table 1**).[25]

MANAGEMENT

Glaucoma management is aimed at reducing IOP, the only modifiable risk factor at this time. The goal fundamentally is to slow or cease structural and functional progression

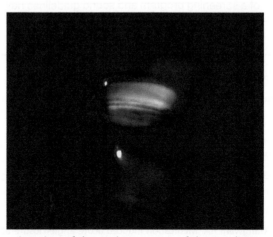

Fig. 5. Gonioscopy prism view of the angle structures of the eye demonstrating trabecular meshwork. (*Courtesy of* Wills Eye Glaucoma Service, Philadelphia, PA; with permission.)

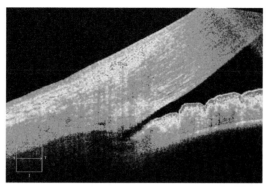

Fig. 6. Anterior segment optical coherence tomography further image of anterior segment structures. (*From* Wills Eye Hospital Diagnostic Center, Philadelphia, PA; with permission.)

of the disease by reducing IOP in several ways (discussed later). In doing so, the real goal is to maintain adequate visual function for an expected life span.

Several studies have clearly established the value of lowering IOP in the management of glaucoma.[9–12] The extent to which IOP should be lowered hinges on the stage of disease. Typically, more aggressive IOP lowering is required in more advanced stages of glaucoma to slow progression. The Collaborative Normal Tension Glaucoma Study established the value for IOP lowering in eyes with glaucoma but with otherwise average IOP.[14] Goals for therapy should be highly individualized based on several factors, including stage at diagnosis, overall health status and projected life span based on comorbidities and age, and highest IOPs in the past. The fundamental goal in glaucoma is to slow down the rate of glaucomatous damage to a point where hopefully as much functional vision as possible is retained.

There are 3 primary modalities of lowering IOP: medical therapy, laser, and surgical modalities. Commonly, early/moderate disease is treated with a combination of medical and laser therapy.[29] Surgical IOP lowering, previously reserved for cases refractory to other less invasive modes of management, has a significantly expanding scope as safety and efficacy of these techniques continues to be enhanced.

Medical Therapy

There are several effective classes of topical therapies for glaucoma. A commonly used class is the topical prostaglandin analogs, which enhance outflow of aqueous humor. These medications are administered once daily with well-established

Table 1 Screening frequency	
Patient Population	**Screening Frequency**
Age 40–60 with no risk factors	3–5 y
Age 40–60 with 1 + risk factors	1–2 y
Age >60	1–2 y

Data from American Academy of Ophthalmology Glaucoma Panel. Preferred Practice Pattern® Guidelines. Primary Open-Angle Glaucoma. San Francisco, CA: American Academy of Ophthalmology; 2010. Available at: www.aao.org/ppp.

efficacy.[30] Typical side effects with this class of medications may include increased eyelash length, potential hyperemia of the conjunctiva, potentially permanent darkening of the iris, and possible attenuation of the periorbital fat.

β-Blockers are another class of medication that reduces aqueous humor formation. A history of chronic obstructive pulmonary disease or asthma is clearly a relative contraindication. Furthermore, caution in patients with cardiac abnormalities/bradyarrhythmias should be used. Carbonic anhydrase inhibitors and α-adrenergic agonists are 2 other classes of medications that reduce aqueous formation and, thereby, are effective for IOP lowering.

As with other common insidious chronic conditions, such as hypertension, the effectiveness of medical therapy is limited by treatment adherence. Because of the dynamic nature of IOP fluctuation and elevation, combined with the lack of any symptomatic reminders by the silent disease itself, regular medical therapy poses a problem for many patients. Additionally, many patients may require multiple drops, which complicates dosing regimens and has a further negative impact on treatment adherence. Given that the preponderance of this disease affects the older population, there are dexterity, proprioceptive, and other issues that may limit a patient's abilities to regularly use these topical therapies.[31]

There are no effective ways of measuring treatment adherence as well. A variety of techniques, such as patient education, reminders, videos, and medication dosing aids, have all been used to attempt to address this subject.

The degree of IOP reduction for an individual patient, like any medical therapy, can vary depending on the effectiveness for that individual counterbalanced with tolerability, which in turn affects adherence (**Table 2**).

Table 2
Ocular antihypertensive classes

Ocular Antihypertensive Class	Mechanism	Intraoclar Pressure Reduction	Side Effects
β-Adrenergic antagonists	↓ Production	20%–25%	Congestive heart failure Bronchospasm Bradycardia Depression Impotence
Prostaglandin analogs	↑ Outflow	25%–33%	Increased eyelash length Conjunctival injection Darkening of iris Attenuation of periorbital fat
Carbonic anhydrase inhibitors	↓ Production	15%–20%	Steven-Johnson Syndrome Malaise Renal calculi
Sympathomimetic agonists	↑ Outflow ↓ Production	20%–25%	Conjunctival injection Fatigue Headache
Parasympathomimetic agents	↑ Outflow	20%–25%	Decreased vision
Hyperosmotics	↑ Blood osmolality	—	Congestive heart failure Urinary retention

Laser

A laser modality in open-angle glaucoma called trabeculoplasty uses laser energy directed at the trabecular meshwork to increase outflow of aqueous humor and thereby lower IOP.

Both the safety and efficacy of this treatment option have been well established and can be used at any point in the treatment plan, either as initial treatment or adjunctive to medical therapies.[32,33] Laser trabeculoplasty also carries great value in nonadherant or medication intolerant patients.

Laser peripheral iridotomy is another type of laser treatment indicated for angle-closure glaucoma. Laser iridotomy entails creating a microscopic opening in the peripheral iris to relieve obstruction of aqueous passage from the posterior to the anterior chambers and enable access to the trabecular meshwork for outflow. Iridotomy may be required for treatment of acute angle-closure glaucoma and also prophylactically in eyes with narrow or crowded anterior chamber angles deemed at risk for developing angle-closure glaucoma in a lifetime.[34]

Surgical

Glaucoma surgical modalities are often used when patients are refractory to medical and/or laser therapies. Traditional surgical modalities hinge on bypassing aqueous humor externally to collect in the subconjunctival space.[35] The trabeculectomy has been well established as a highly effective method of substantial IOP lowering (**Fig. 7**). This procedure involves creating a partial thickness scleral flap under which a fistula is made into the anterior chamber. This enables guarded percolation of the aqueous humor to the subconjunctival space in a region, termed a *bleb*, for recirculation.

Chemotherapeutic antimetabolites are applied typically to enhance success rates because long-term IOP lowering hinges on limiting patient fibrosis in the region of this surgically created drain.[36]

Tube shunts represent synthetic devices that shunt fluid to a reservoir (**Fig. 8**). The safety and efficacy of tube shunts have been well established and have a strong role in eyes with prior scarring or prior surgeries or in some cases as primary procedures.

Additional smaller incision glaucoma surgical techniques are more recently emerging because new devices are both in development and currently used to

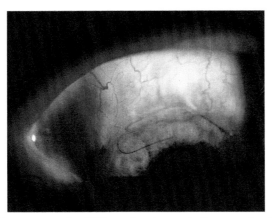

Fig. 7. Trabeculectomy surgery for IOP lowering demonstrating a conjunctival filtering bleb (diversion of aqueous fluid traversing under a scleral flap.). (*Courtesy of* Wills Eye Glaucoma Service, Philadelphia, PA; with permission.)

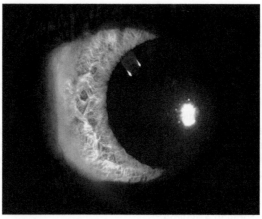

Fig. 8. Tube shunt inserted to divert aqueous fluid to an extraocular reservoir implanted into the subconjunctival space. (*Courtesy of* Wills Eye Glaucoma Service, Philadelphia, PA; with permission.)

achieve IOP lowering with greater safety profiles while keeping traditional surgical modalities as options in the future. Currently, these techniques are reserved for eyes with earlier/moderate stage disease.

Future Therapy

There are several exciting areas for glaucoma treatment that are being actively explored. From a diagnostic standpoint, earlier detection in higher-risk populations through telemedicine as imaging devices improve quality and sensitivity holds promise. From a medical treatment standpoint, new IOP-lowering topical agents are in various phases of clinical trials.[37,38] Different modes of drug delivery that may reduce a patient's dependence on self-administration may improve overall outcomes directly addressing concerns of treatment adherence. The development of a variety of surgical techniques and devices through smaller incisions enabling quicker visual rehabilitation with a lower risk profile is emerging as well.

Monitoring and Follow-up

Patients with glaucoma should be actively monitored at regular frequent intervals by an ophthalmologist. Management of glaucoma is a lifelong process. The frequency hinges on the stage of the disease and stability. Any patient with known risk factors should be referred for a comprehensive ophthalmologic evaluation.[39,40]

SUMMARY

Glaucoma is a significant global health problem that affects 67 million people worldwide. It is the second leading cause of blindness both in the United States and worldwide and the world's commonest cause of irreversible blindness. Glaucoma is a multifactorial degenerative optic neuropathy that can progress at variable rates and can afflict all age groups, for which elevated IOP is a major modifiable risk factor.

The disease can be characterized into 2 major subtypes based on the status of the internal drainage system: open angle and angle closure. In open-angle glaucoma, the drainage system demonstrates no evident obstruction but is functionally and structurally deficient, leading typically to elevated IOP. Risk factors for open-angle glaucoma include family history, increased IOP, older age (>60), increased cup-to-disc ratio, and thinner central corneas. Angle-closure glaucoma can present acutely with symptoms of pain, decreased vision, and nausea, or chronically without symptoms and represents closure of the internal drainage system typically due to obstruction by the peripheral iris. Risk factors for angle-closure glaucoma include hyperopia (smaller eye), older age, female gender, and Asian ethnicity.

Glaucoma is a clinical diagnosis, based on characteristic optic nerve changes associated with corresponding visual field deficits, regardless of IOP. IOP lowering has been shown in robust trials to meaningfully slow the rate of glaucoma progression. Management of glaucoma can include topical and oral medical therapies, laser modalities, and surgical management all aimed at lowering IOP. Patients with any risk factors for glaucoma should be referred to an ophthalmologist for a comprehensive evaluation.

REFERENCES

1. Quigley HA. Number of people with glaucoma worldwide. Br J Ophthalmol 1996; 80:389–93.
2. Quigley HA, Vitale S. Models of open-angle glaucoma prevalence and incidence in the United States. Invest Ophthalmol Vis Sci 1997;38:83–91.
3. The Eye Disease Research Group. Prevalence of open-angle glaucoma among adults in the United States. Arch Ophthalmol 2004;122:532–8.
4. Distelhorst JS, Hughes GM. Open-angle glaucoma. Am Fam Physician 2003; 67(9):1937–44.
5. Sommer A, Tielsch JM, Katz J, et al. Racial differences in the cause-specific prevalence of blindness in east Baltimore. N Engl J Med 1991;325:1412–7.
6. Tielsch JM, Sommer A, Katz J, et al. Racial variations in the prevalence of primary open-angle glaucoma. The Baltimore Eye Survey. JAMA 1991;266:369–74.
7. Hyams S. Angle-closure glaucoma: a comprehensive review of primary and secondary angle-closure glaucoma. Amsterdam: Kugler & Ghedini; 1990.
8. Quigley HA, Broman AT. The number of people with glaucoma worldwide in 2010 and 2020. Br J Ophthalmol 2006;90:262–7.
9. Gordon MO, Kass MA. The Ocular Hypertension Treatment Study: design and baseline description of the participants. Arch Ophthalmol 1999;117:573–83.
10. Leske MC, Heijl A, Hyman L, et al. Early Manifest Glaucoma Trial: design and baseline data. Ophthalmology 1999;106:2144–53.
11. Musch DC, Lichter PR, Guire KE, et al. The Collaborative Initial Glaucoma Treatment Study: study design, methods, and baseline characteristics of enrolled patients. Ophthalmology 1999;106:653–62.
12. Ederer F, Gaasterland DE, Sullivan EK, et al. The Advanced Glaucoma Intervention Study (AGIS): 1. Study design and methods and baseline characteristics of study patients. Control Clin Trials 1994;15:299–325.
13. Summaries for patients. Screening for glaucoma: U.S. Preventive Services Task Force recommendation statement. Ann Intern Med 2013;159(7):1.
14. Anderson DR. Collaborative normal tension glaucoma study. Curr Opin Ophthalmol 2003;14:86–90.
15. Nolan WP, Foster PJ, Devereux JG, et al. YAG laser iridotomy treatment for primary angleclosure in east Asian eyes. Br J Ophthalmol 2000;84:1255–9.
16. Gazzard G, Friedman DS, Devereux JG, et al. A prospective ultrasound biomicroscopy evaluation of changes in anterior segment morphology after laser iridotomy in Asian eyes. Ophthalmology 2003;110:630–8.
17. Fontana SC, Brubaker RF. Volume and depth of the anterior chamber in the normal aging human eye. Arch Ophthalmol 1980;98:1803–8.

18. Racette L, Wilson MR, Zangwill LM, et al. Primary open-angle glaucoma in blacks: a review. Surv Ophthalmol 2003;48(3):295–313.
19. Tielsch JM, Katz J, Sommer A, et al. Family history and risk of primary open angle glaucoma. The Baltimore Eye Survey. Arch Ophthalmol 1994;112(1):69–73.
20. Foster PJ, Alsbirk PH, Baasanhu J, et al. Anterior chamber depth in Mongolians. Variation with age, sex and method of measurement. Am J Ophthalmol 1997;124:53–60.
21. Coffi GA, Durcan FJ, Girkin CA, et al. Angle Closure Glaucoma. Chapter 5 in Section 10 of Basic and clinical science course 2008–2009. Am Acad Ophthalmol 2008;5:126–8.
22. Yamamoto T, Iwase A, Araie M, et al. The Tajimi Study report 2: prevalence of primary angle closure and secondary glaucoma in a Japanese population. Ophthalmology 2005;112:1661–9.
23. Traverso CE, Bagnis A, Bricola G. Angle-closure glaucoma. In: Yanoff M, Duker J, editors. Ophthalmology. 2nd edition. St. Louis (MO): Mosby; 2004. p. 1491–8.
24. American Academy of Ophthalmology. Primary angle closure glaucoma, preferred practice pattern. San Francisco: American Academy of Ophthalmology; 2010. Available at: www.aao.org/ppp http://one.aao.org/preferred-practice-pattern/primary-angle-closure-ppp–october-2010. Accessed August 14, 2014.
25. American Academy of Ophthalmology. Primary open angle glaucoma, preferred practice pattern. San Francisco: American Academy of Ophthalmology; 2010. Available at: www.aao.org/ppp http://one.aao.org/preferred-practice-pattern/primary-openangle-glaucoma-ppp–october-2010. Accessed 14 Aug 2014.
26. Harper R, Reeves B. The sensitivity and specificity of direct ophthalmoscopic optic disc assessment in screening for glaucoma: a multivariate analysis. Graefes Arch Clin Exp Ophthalmol 2000;238(12):949–55.
27. Martus P, Stroux A, Budde WM, et al. Predictive factors for progressive optic nerve damage in various types of chronic open-angle glaucoma. Am J Ophthalmol 2005;139:999–1009.
28. Barkana Y, Dorairaj SK, Gerber Y, et al. Agreement between gonioscopy and ultrasound biomicroscopy in detecting iridotrabecular apposition. Arch Ophthalmol 2007;125:1331–5.
29. Singh K, Lee BL, Wilson R, on behalf of the glaucoma modified RAND-like Methodology Group. A panel assessment of glaucoma management: modification of existing RAND-like methodology for consensus in ophthalmology. Part II: results and interpretation. Am J Ophthalmol 2008;145(3):575–81.
30. Migdal C, Gregory W, Hitchings R. Long-term functional outcome after early surgery compared with laser and medicine in open angle glaucoma. Ophthalmology 1994;101(10):1651–6.
31. Osterberg L, Blaschke T. Adherence to medication. N Engl J Med 2005;353:487–97.
32. The Glaucoma Laser Trial (GLT) and glaucoma laser trial follow-up study: 7. Results. Glaucoma Laser Trial Research Group. Am J Ophthalmol 1995;120:718–31.
33. The AGIS Investigators. The Advanced Glaucoma Intervention Study (AGIS) 13. Comparison of treatment outcomes within race: 10-year results. Ophthalmology 2004;111:651–64.
34. Lowe RF. Acute angle-closure glaucoma. The second eye: an analysis of 200 cases. Br J Ophthalmol 1962;46:641–50.
35. Cairns JE. Trabeculectomy. Preliminary report of a new method. Am J Ophthalmol 1968;66(4):673–9.
36. Suzuki R, Dickens CJ, Iwach AG, et al. Long-term follow-up of initially successful trabeculectomy with 5-fluorouracil injections. Ophthalmology 2002;109:1921–4.

37. Epstein DL. Open angle glaucoma. Why not a cure? Arch Ophthalmol 1987; 105(9):1187–8.
38. Rao PV, Deng PF, Kumar J, et al. Modulation of aqueous humor outflow facility by the Rho kinasespecific inhibitor Y-27632. Invest Ophthalmol Vis Sci 2001;42(5): 1029–37.
39. Hennis A, Wu S-Y, Nemesure B, et al. Awareness of incident open-angle glaucoma in a population study. The Barbados Eye Studies. Ophthalmology 2007; 114(10):1816–21.
40. Leske MC, Wu SY, Honkanen R, et al. Nine-year incidence of open-angle glaucoma in the Barbados Eye Studies. Ophthalmology 2007;114(6):1058–64.

Diabetic Retinopathy

Andrew M. Hendrick, MD[a],*, Maria V. Gibson, MD, PhD[b],
Ambar Kulshreshtha, MD, PhD, MPH[b]

KEYWORDS

- Diabetic retinopathy • Nonproliferative diabetic retinopathy
- Proliferative diabetic retinopathy • Glycemic control • Visual impairment

KEY POINTS

- Diabetic retinopathy (DR) is a microvascular complication of diabetes and is a leading cause of vision loss and visual disability in working-age adults.
- Blindness due to DR can be prevented with adequate screening and treatment.
- Patients with diabetes without evidence of DR can have their eyes examined every 2 years. Patients at high risk (long duration of diabetes, poor glycemic and lipid control, and hypertension) require an annual eye examination.
- Nonmydriatic single 45° field cost-effective retinal photography has adequate sensitivity, specificity, and low technical failure rate to detect DR.
- Treatment includes intensive management of diabetes, laser, intravitreal medication delivery, and surgery.

INTRODUCTION

Diabetic retinopathy (DR) is a common microvascular complication of diabetes. With increasing global prevalence of diabetes, DR is a major cause of vision impairment affecting approximately 4.2 million people worldwide.[1] The number of Americans 40 years or older with DR is estimated to reach 16.0 million by 2050, with vision-threatening diabetic retinopathy affecting an estimated 3.4 million of them. DR is a major public health burden with direct medical costs accounting for $492 million, in addition to lost time and wages associated with receiving care.[2] The focus of this article is to review salient features of DR, including pathophysiology, screening, and treatment.

DEFINITION

DR is the clinically visible manifestation of longstanding diabetes in the ocular fundus. Its presence reflects the combination of longevity of disease duration and degree of

Nothing to disclose.
[a] Department of Ophthalmology, Emory University, Emory Eye Center, 1365B Clifton Road, Atlanta, GA 30322, USA; [b] Department of Family Medicine, Emory University, Emory Family Medicine Center, 4500 Shallowford Road, Dunwoody, GA 30338, USA
* Corresponding author.
E-mail address: ahendrick@emory.edu

glycemic control. Although good systemic control of blood pressure and blood sugar will delay onset and progression, DR will affect nearly all patients with sufficient duration of disease.[3,4] This disease progresses through predictable stepwise stages, categorically moving from the initial nonproliferative type to the more advanced, proliferative type. Ophthalmoscopic features of DR are summarized in **Box 1** and **Fig. 1**.

Nonproliferative DR (NPDR) is characterized by the presence of aneurysms, hemorrhages, exudation, and other abnormalities in the retinal circulation. These microvascular features are commonly found in other conditions that can affect retinal circulation and can be distinguished with knowledge of the patient's history (**Box 2**).

The critical distinction separating NPDR and proliferative DR (PDR) is the presence of ocular neovascularization. Ocular neovascularization is most commonly found in the iris, in the retina, or at the optic nerve and represents a significant threat to vision even with treatment. Specific classification of DR is summarized in **Box 3**.

Pathophysiology of Diabetic Retinopathy

Several biomechanical pathways have been proposed that link hyperglycemia to microvascular complications, including formation of advanced glycated end products,

---

Box 1
Features of diabetic retinopathy

- *Microaneurysms*: small circular red lesions in the retina; represents saccular vascular weakness and typical focal point of vascular leakage, represents early signs of DR (see **Fig. 1**)

- *Intraretinal hemorrhages*: larger, more irregular red lesions in the retina; not intrinsically visually threatening, generally resolve within 3 to 4 months (**Fig. 2**)

- *Hard exudates*: yellow irregular shaped lesions; represent intraretinal lipids and protein deposition. When accompanied by retinal thickening, represent feature of diabetic macular edema (**Fig. 3**)

- *Cotton-wool spots*: superficial feather-bordered white lesions; represent nerve fiber layer infarctions from capillary occlusion (**Fig. 4**)

- *Intraretinal microvascular abnormalities*: alterations to blood vessel from capillary closure that lead to visible vascular remodeling

- *Venous beading*: dilated, tortuous, and irregular in caliber veins adjacent to capillary nonperfusion

- *Macular edema*[a]: breakdown of the blood-retinal barrier promotes leakage of plasma from bloodstream into the retina causing swelling; can occur early in DR development, often presents alongside hard exudates and microaneurysms (see **Fig. 3**)

- *Neovascularization*[a]: fine, lacy abnormal proliferation of new blood vessels; can extend into the vitreous cavity and hemorrhage into the vitreous (**Fig. 5**)

- *Vitreous hemorrhage*[a]: bleeding into the vitreous cavity (see **Fig. 5**)

- *Tractional retinal detachment*[a]: contraction of fibrous proliferation associated with neovascularization can separate the retina from its anatomic position

- *Neovascular glaucoma*[a]: new blood vessel growth into the eye's drainage system occludes it, driving up intraocular pressure

[a] Vision threatening.
From Early treatment diabetic retinopathy study design and baseline patient characteristics. Ophthalmology 1991;98(Suppl 5):741–56; with permission.

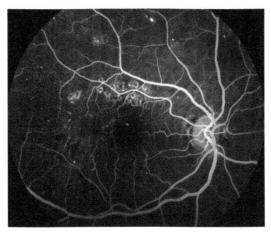

Fig. 1. Fluorescein angiogram, right eye, transit phase. Multiple light-bulb microaneurysms are visibly hyperfluorescent in the macula alongside the visible laser burns in the superior macula.

oxidative stress, polyol accumulation, and activation of protein kinase C. The pathways modulate the disease process through effects on cellular metabolism, signaling, and growth factors. These processes lead to the development of microvascular damage, increased capillary permeability, vascular occlusion, and weakening of supporting structures as a result of hyperglycemia. With longer duration of the disease, chronic hyperglycemia damages the retinal blood vessels and pericytes are lost, leading to involution of the vascular changes in microcirculation and loss of normal capillary exchange and promoting leakage of endovascular products.[5,6] Hypoxia advances upregulation of vascular endothelial growth factor (VEGF) platelet adhesiveness, erythrocyte aggregation, serum lipids, and fibrinolysis. VEGF is an important contributor to both vascular leakage and promotion of new blood vessel growth and forms the basis of treatment of vision-threatening disease.[7]

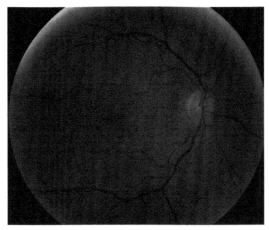

Fig. 2. Fundus photograph, right eye. Numerous punctate red circular microaneurysms are visible. A large dot blot hemorrhage is adjacent to a branch of the inferotemporal arcade.

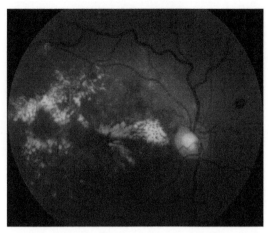

Fig. 3. Fundus photograph, right eye. Massive intraretinal lipid exudation and retinal thickening within the macula from DME.

Epidemiology

Much of the understanding regarding the epidemiology of DR is derived from the Wisconsin Epidemiologic Study of Diabetic Retinopathy data. This study was a population-based study performed more than 30 years ago in a predominantly racially white region. The study formed the basis of several treatment principles that still apply. After 20 years of follow-up, 99% of patients with type 1 diabetes and 60% with type 2 diabetes have some degree of DR.[3]

The epidemiology of diabetes mellitus (DM) and DR is evolving as prevalence rates increase. A 2008 NHANES (National Health and Nutrition Examination Survey) survey of US adults over 40 years old estimated that 28% of people with diabetes have DR and 4% have vision-threatening disease. Notably, this study demonstrated racial

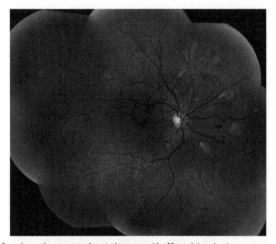

Fig. 4. Montage fundus photograph, right eye. Fluffy white lesions scattered in superficial retina surround the optic nerve. An intraretinal microvascular abnormality can be found in the superonasal fundus.

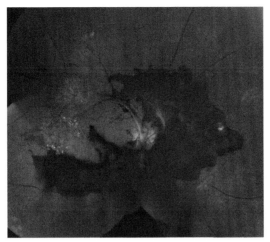

Fig. 5. Montage fundus photograph, right eye. Vitreous hemorrhage and neovascularization of the nerve and elsewhere are visible in this patient with proliferative DR.

disparities as well such that non-Hispanic black individuals had higher rates of DR and vision-threatening DR (38.8% and 5.9%, respectively).[8] Risk factors for development of DR are summarized in **Box 4**.

Symptoms

It should be noted that retinopathy is not the only visually threatening aspect of diabetic ocular disease. Individuals with DM also have increased risk of cataracts and cranial neuropathies, which can lead to visual blurring or double vision, respectively.

Box 2
Systemic and ocular disorders that may mimic diabetic retinopathy

Systemic disorders that may mimic DR

    Hypertension

    Obstructive sleep apnea

    Chronic kidney disease

    Sickle cell disease

    Anemia

    Systemic infections

    Vasculitis

Ocular disorders that may mimic DR

    Retinal vein occlusion

    Radiation retinopathy

    Macular telangiectasia

    Ocular ischemic syndrome

From Ryan SJ, Schachat AP, Wilkinson CP, et al. Retina. 5th edition. Elsevier; 2013; with permission.

Box 3
Classification of diabetic retinopathy

Mild nonproliferative diabetic retinopathy

- Microaneurysms

Moderate nonproliferative diabetic retinopathy

- Intraretinal hemorrhages, hard exudates, cotton wool spots, venous beading less than required for severe nonproliferative diabetic retinopathy

Severe nonproliferative diabetic retinopathy

Any of the following (4/2/1 rule)

- Extensive intraretinal hemorrhages in each of 4 quadrants
- Venous beading in more than 2 quadrants
- One intraretinal microvascular abnormality

Proliferative diabetic retinopathy

Any of the following

- Neovascularization
- Vitreous/preretinal hemorrhage

From Canadian Ophthalmological Society. Canadian Ophthalmological Society evidence-based clinical practice guidelines for the management of diabetic retinopathy. Can J Ophthalmol 2012;47:1–30; with permission.

Intrinsically, DR does not cause symptoms, especially if only one eye is affected (which leads to problems for screening compliance). The causes of blindness from DR are diabetic macular edema (DME) and PDR, which are discussed later.

Diabetic macular edema

The macula is the anatomic center of the retina and contains the area responsible for highest visual potential. DME is the presence of retinal thickening within the center of vision, and when present, can lead to blurring and distortion of vision, representing the most frequent cause of vision loss from DR. It can occur at any stage of DR. Clinically, DME appears as blunting of the retinal contour, hard exudates, and visible retinal

---

Box 4
Risk factors associated with the development and progression of diabetic retinopathy

- Duration of diabetes
- Type 1 diabetes
- Poor diabetes control
- Poor blood pressure control
- Hyperlipidemia
- Nephropathy
- Pregnancy
- Hispanic and African American race

Data from Refs.[9–14]

---

thickening. Treatments have emerged within the past decade that greatly enhance the potential to regain eyesight when it has become impaired.[10]

Proliferative diabetic retinopathy
Advancement from NPDR to PDR is defined by the presence of new blood vessels, or neovascularization. Perhaps counterintuitively, the presence of neovascularization in response to chronic hypoxia is not a helpful adaptation and is associated with a poor visual prognosis when unchecked. Vision is lost in this most advanced form of DR from vitreous hemorrhage and tractional retinal detachment.

Vitreous hemorrhage
New blood vessel growth into the vitreous from the retina can spontaneously shear, leading to spillage of blood into the vitreous cavity. This blood manifests as black debris, shadows, and floaters in the vision. If sufficiently dense, a vitreous hemorrhage can diminish visual acuity from mildly impaired to unable to see movement. Vision loss from a vitreous hemorrhage can however be restored with resolution of the hemorrhage.

Tractional retinal detachment
Neovascularization does not occur in isolation. Accompanying fibrous and glial support tissue has contractile properties. This fibrovascular proliferation can engage the retina with enough force to separate it from the underlying tissues, causing it to detach. Detachment of the retina can lead to irreversible vision loss unless successful surgical repair is enacted within a reasonable timeframe.

Diagnostic Modalities

Laboratory studies of hemoglobin A_{1c} (HbA$_{1c}$) levels are important in the long-term follow-up care of patients with diabetes and DR. Monitoring of other sequelae of diabetes is also very important and should include analysis of kidney function, microalbuminuria, lipid levels, foot examinations, and assessments of the peripheral nerve function. Specific ocular tools are summarized in **Table 1**.

Management of Diabetic Retinopathy

Optimization of systemic well-being in patients with DM is a fundamental concept whose importance cannot be overstated. Blood pressure, lipid management, and blood sugar control form the basis for not only long-term survival but also protection

Table 1 Ocular imaging tools	
Fundus photography	• Excellent for capturing funduscopic characteristics as a baseline • Clinical teaching tool to engage patients in their care
Optical coherence tomography	• Provides 2-dimensional cross-sectional view of macular anatomy • Allows quantitative analysis of the thickness of the retina to diagnose any DME, or retinal detachment • Is an essential tool to manage anti-VEGF therapy
Fluorescein angiography	• Provides exquisite detailed view of en face retinal vascular anatomy • Allows determination of pinpoint microaneurysms, allowing targeting during laser photocoagulation • Permits visualization of extent of capillary nonperfusion and neovascularization, when present
B-scan ultrasonography	• Helpful when vitreous hemorrhage precludes adequate visualization of the fundus

From Ryan SJ, Schachat AP, Wilkinson CP, et al. Retina. 5th edition. Elsevier; 2013; with permission.

from worsening eye disease. DR management should be guided by evidence-based recommendations regarding risk stratification and appropriate referral, modalities for examination, frequency of follow-ups, and interventions for treatment.

Early detection of DR relies on educating patients with diabetes about the importance of a comprehensive eye examination and timely intervention even though the patient may be asymptomatic (**Box 5**). The recommended screening modality for DR is a dilated slit lamp biomicroscopy with a lens or dilated fundoscopy, including stereoscopic examination of the posterior pole by an ophthalmologist or optometrist. Use of new technologies such as digital cameras and teleophthalmology can improve access to screening. A nonmydriatic single 45° field retinal photography has adequate sensitivity, specificity, and low technical failure rate to detect DR. Grading by an offsite ophthalmologist can make this a cost-effective option. Imaging technology, however, does not mitigate the need for comprehensive eye examinations to identify other DM eye complications including cataract and glaucoma.

Management Goals

Glucose control

Glycemic control is the major modifiable risk factor for reduced risk in both onset and progression of DR. For every percentage point decrease in HbA_{1c} (eg, from 8% to 7%)

Box 5
Diabetic retinopathy screening recommendations

- For individuals with type 1 diabetes diagnosed after puberty, screening for DR should be initiated 5 years after the diagnosis of diabetes.

- For individuals diagnosed with type 1 diabetes before puberty, screening for DR should be initiated at puberty, unless there are other considerations that would suggest the need for an earlier examination.

- Screening for DR in individuals with type 2 diabetes should be initiated at the time of diagnosis of diabetes.

- Subsequent screening for DR in individuals depends on the level of retinopathy.

  a. In those who do not show evidence of retinopathy, screening should occur every year.

  b. In those with type 1 diabetes, every 1 to 2 years; in those with type 2 diabetes, should be determined by anticipated compliance.

  c. Once NPDR is detected, examination should be conducted at least annually for mild NPDR, or more frequently (at 3- to 6-month intervals) for moderate or severe DR.

  d. For severe NPDR, PDR and clinically significant macular edema, examination usually conducted every 2 to 4 months.

- For diabetes diagnosed before pregnancy, conduct a comprehensive eye examination during the first trimester of pregnancy.

  a. If there is minimal DR or mild to moderate NPDR, a 3- to 12-month follow-up interval is recommended.

  b. For severe NPDR or worse, 1- to 3-month interval is recommended.

  c. Ophthalmic review and treatment need to be performed expeditiously (typically within 1–4 weeks) for patients with PDR and macular edema.

Data from Canadian Ophthalmological Society. Canadian Ophthalmological Society evidence-based clinical practice guidelines for the management of diabetic retinopathy. Can J Ophthalmol 2012;47:1–30; and ADA. Standards of medical care in diabetes–2014. Diabetes Care 2014;37(Suppl 1):S14–80.

in patients with type 2 diabetes, there can be up to a 35% reduction in the risk of microvascular complications.[4] The results of the Diabetes Control and Complications Trial, a multicenter randomized control study, demonstrated that over a 6.5-year follow-up, intensive glycemic control (median HbA$_{1c}$: 7.3%) with conventional (median HbA$_{1c}$: 9.1%) treatment was associated with reduction in any DR by 76% and progression of DR by 54%.[15]

Similarly, the United Kingdom Prospective Diabetes Study (UKPDS) study demonstrated that intensive treatment reduced the development of any DR by 25% and showed a 29% reduction in progression to requirement of laser photocoagulation in the intensive group compared with conventional treatment.[16]

Blood pressure control

Optimization of blood pressure in patients with hypertension is a major factor in reducing the progression of DR. In the UKPDS, tight blood pressure control with the use of an angiotensin-converting enzyme inhibitor or a β-blocker had a 34% reduction in progression of retinopathy and a 47% reduced risk of deterioration in visual acuity of 3 lines in association with a 10/5 mm Hg reduction in blood pressure.[4] However, a 4-year follow-up from the ACCORD (Action to Control Cardiovascular Risk in Diabetes Trial) Eye study blood pressure trial demonstrated that there was no significant difference in the progression of DR with intensive (target systolic BP: <120 mm Hg) versus standard BP control (target systolic BP: <140 mm Hg) in patients with type 2 DM.[16]

Lipid control

Observational studies suggest that dyslipidemia increases the risk of DR, particularly DME.[11] In the Fenofibrate Intervention and Event Lowering in Diabetes (FIELD) study, among patients with type 2 diabetes, those treated with fenofibrate were less likely than controls to need laser treatment (5.2% vs 3.6%).[17] The Early Treatment of Diabetic Retinopathy Study data suggest that lipid lowering may also decrease the risk of hard exudate formation and associated vision loss in patients with DR.[18] Other management goals are described in **Table 2**.

Treatment modalities are described in **Table 3**.

PHARMACOLOGIC STRATEGIES
Systemic Medications

Aspirin

In the ETDRS (Early Treatment Diabetic Retinopathy Study), aspirin (650 mg/d) was shown to have no effect on retinopathy or vitreous hemorrhage. As a result, primary care physicians can feel comfortable that there are no ocular contraindications to the use of aspirin when required for cardiovascular disease (CVD) or other medical indications.[24]

Fenofibrate

Fenofibrate is a medication used for hypercholesterolemia that likely has more ancillary benefits than is currently understood. Use of fenofibrate in 2 large independent clinical trials (FIELD and ACCORD) demonstrated a reduced risk of retinopathy progression.[16,17] Unless contraindications exist, the addition of fenofibrate to the therapeutic regimen should be considered.

Ocular Medications

Medication can be injected directly into the vitreous via a procedure in the clinic by retinal specialists. This medication offers direct benefit of delivery to the tissue of interest with minimal systemic exposure. Intravitreal injections require sterile technique

Table 2
Diabetic retinopathy management goals

Factors	Mechanism	Management Goals
Blood glucose[18,19]	Continuous relationship between A1C and microvascular complications. Impacts other sites within the eye including the lens, anterior chamber, and iris. Intensive control reduces risk of development and rate of progression of DR.	• Initiate tight control of blood glucose early in the course of DM • Target A1C <7.0% except in older adults or those with comorbid conditions • Adjust A1C in individuals at risk of hypoglycemia • In patients aged 0–6, 6–12, and 13–19 years, use patient age as a consideration in the establishment of glycemic goals for type 1 diabetes, with different targets for preprandial, bedtime/overnight, and HbA$_{1c}$ levels
Hypertension[16,19]	Blood pressure control reduces risk of development and rate of progression of DR and risk of vitreous hemorrhage. Also has a positive impact on other diabetic complications.	• Treat to achieve optimal control of BP <140/90 mm Hg • Diastolic BP may be a better predictor of progression of DR
Dyslipidemia[11,17–19]	Hyperlipidemia associated with exudative maculopathy, DME, and vision loss	• Target low-density lipoprotein <100 mg/dL • Statins may slow the progression of retinopathy • Fenofibrate reduces risk of DR progression
Smoking[20,21]	Increases the risk of DR, nephropathy, and neuropathy and other macrovascular complications.	Smoking cessation is important to reduce the risk of CVD, effect on DR remains controversial
Exercise[19,22]	High impact may exacerbate vitreous hemorrhage in patients with PDR.	Exercise prescriptions improved psychological well-being and participation in daily activities. Caution is suggested for high-impact striating, anaerobic exercise in patients with PDR
Pregnancy[14,23]	Increased risk of rapid progression of DR.	Initiate eye examination before pregnancy, during each trimester, and within the first year postpartum

Data from Refs.[11,14,16–23]

and carry low but important risk of complications, such as retinal detachment and severe infection. Furthermore, the effect of the medications is temporary, and the injections frequently need to be repeated monthly.

Intravitreal anti-vascular endothelial growth factor therapy (bevacizumab, ranibizumab, aflibercept, pegaptanib)

VEGF is upregulated by conditions of poor blood flow, and anti-VEGF therapy provides the foundation for therapy for visually threatening diabetic eye disease. As a

Table 3
Diabetic retinopathy treatment modalities

Treatment	Mechanism	Implications
Antiplatelet therapy/aspirin[24]	Decreases platelet activation and aggregation. Decreases prostaglandin production.	Antiplatelet therapy, including aspirin, has not shown any demonstrable effect on the progression of DR, may be required for concomitant CVD.
Antiangiogenic agents (VEGF inhibitors) (Bevacizumab, Ranibizumab)[25,26]	Inhibits angiogenesis and induces rapid regression of neovascularization.	Intravitreal administration has shown benefit in regression of PDR and resolution of DME.
Intraocular corticosteroids[27]	Modulation of inflammatory response. Inhibits PG release, inhibits cellular proliferation, and stabilizes neovascularization.	Triamcinolone administered intravitreally is occasionally used in treatment of DME.
Laser photocoagulation (focal vs panretinal)[24]	PRP is the preferred form of treatment of PDR. It involves applying laser burns over the entire retina, sparing the central macular area. Focal laser involves delivery of laser burns within the macula for DME.	The presence of high-risk PDR is an indication for immediate treatment. Patients may experience field loss and macular edema after PRP. Visual potential of laser is less robust than intravitreal anti-VEGF therapy but still has distinct clinical utility.
Vitrectomy[28]	Removes vitreous to clear nonclearing vitreous hemorrhage or repair detached retina.	In cases of vitreous hemorrhage, early vitrectomy may result in a slightly greater recovery of vision in patients with type I diabetes.

Data from Refs.[24–28]

class, intravitreal injections of anti-VEGF medications have a multiplicity of beneficial effects:

- Stabilization the blood retinal barrier and reduction in leakage of vascular contents into the retina. Repeated periodic use of intravitreal anti-VEGF injections forms the present standard of care for treatment of DME.
- Rapidly induced regression of active ocular neovascularization. This property is useful adjunctively for treatment of neovascular glaucoma and adjunctively before vitrectomy surgery to reduce intraocular hemorrhage.[25]
- Direct benefit of ameliorating the level of retinopathy. However, this has less clinical utility given that the risk-benefit ratio of serial intravitreal injections does not clearly support this property as distinctly important at this time.[26]

NONPHARMACOLOGIC STRATEGIES
Laser Photocoagulation

Laser has been used for decades in the treatment of advanced DR and involves directing a high-focused beam of light energy to burn the retina and supporting tissues.

Laser photocoagulation is applied for 2 different aspects of DR that vary in the technique of application.

1. Focal laser treatment involves delivery of laser burns within the macula for individuals with DME. During this technique, laser is applied to leaking microaneurysms and to areas of retinal thickening. This treatment has distinct clinical utility in many circumstances, but does not have the same robust potential for visual improvement when compared with anti-VEGF therapy.
2. Panretinal photocoagulation (PRP) is used in the treatment of PDR. It involves applying laser burns over the entire peripheral retina, sparing the macula. This treatment reduces the risk of significant vision loss by 50% of patients for whom it is indicated.[29]

Vitrectomy

Vitrectomy involves surgical removal of the vitreous gel and can typically be performed as outpatient surgery. The main indications for vitrectomy in individuals with PDR are to clear a nonclearing vitreous hemorrhage and repair tractional retinal detachment. The surgeries are highly complex and typically require a prolonged period of time for visual recovery. Treatment modalities are described in **Table 3**.

SPECIAL CIRCUMSTANCE: NEOVASCULAR GLAUCOMA

Severe retinal ischemia can cause new blood vessel development on the surface of the iris, or neovascularization of the iris (NVI). NVI is uniquely challenging to treat because of the potential for increased intraocular pressure (IOP), microcystic edema of the cornea, and damage to the optic nerve. Initial treatment is to lower IOP with topical medications as well as systemic carbonic anhydrase inhibitors or osmotic agents. In patients with DR and NVI, VEGF inhibitor injections can be used in conjunction with PRP to regress the neovascularization and reduce the risk of long-term glaucoma.

Diagnosis and Treatment of Diabetic Retinopathy During Pregnancy

The use of cyclopentolate or tropicamide for pupillary dilation and the use of topical anesthetic drops and fluorescein are safe to use during pregnancy for diagnostic purposes. Fluorescein angiography can be deferred until delivery and breast-feeding. Laser treatment poses no known risk to the fetus. The risk of using VEGF agents during pregnancy is unclear and should be avoided.

CRITERIA FOR URGENT REFERRAL TO AN OPHTHALMOLOGIST

Any sudden severe vision loss or symptoms of retinal detachment in patients with diabetes require same-day referral to an ophthalmologist. Severe NPDR, PDR, and DME NVI are considered vision-threatening retinopathy and warrant prompt evaluation. The presence of any proliferative retinopathy or preretinal or vitreous hemorrhage warrants urgent ophthalmology referral.[30]

SUMMARY

DR is an increasingly common source of vision loss that affects working-age adults. The consequences of undetected and untreated disease can be devastating. Optimal treatment involves intensive systemic management with glycemic control and blood pressure management. Prevention of vision loss relies on early detection and coordination between primary care and ophthalmology. Timely referrals of individuals at greatest risk can have profound benefit in maintenance of activities of daily living.

REFERENCES

1. ADA. National Diabetes Statistics Report, 2014. 2014. http://www.diabetes.org/diabetes-basics/statistics/. Accessed October 2, 2014.
2. Saaddine JB, Honeycutt AA, Narayan KM, et al. Projection of diabetic retinopathy and other major eye diseases among people with diabetes mellitus: United States, 2005-2050. Arch Ophthalmol 2008;126(12):1740–7.
3. Klein R, Klein BE, Moss SE, et al. The Wisconsin Epidemiologic Study of Diabetic Retinopathy. II. Prevalence and risk of diabetic retinopathy when age at diagnosis is less than 30 years. Arch Ophthalmol 1984;102:520–6.
4. Tight blood pressure control and risk of macrovascular and microvascular complications in type 2 diabetes. UK Prospective Diabetes Study Group. BMJ 1998; 317:708–13.
5. Bandello F, Lattanzio R, Zucchiatti I, et al. Pathophysiology and treatment of diabetic retinopathy. Acta Diabetol 2013;50(1):1–20.
6. Antonetti DA, Klein R, Gardner TW. Mechanisms of disease diabetic retinopathy. N Engl J Med 2012;366:1227–39.
7. Tarr JM, Kaul K, Chopra M, et al. Pathophysiology of diabetic retinopathy. Ophthalmology 2013;2013:1–13.
8. Zhang X, Saadine J, Chou CF, et al. Prevalence of diabetic retinopathy in the U.S 2004-2008. JAMA 2010;204(6):649–56.
9. NIH National Eye Institute. Diabetic eye disease, statistics and data [NEI]. 2010. Available at: https://www.nei.nih.gov/eyedata/diabetic.asp. Accessed September 26, 2014.
10. Early Treatment Diabetic Retinopathy Study Research Group. Photocoagulation for diabetic macular edema. Early Treatment Diabetic Retinopathy Study Report Number 1. Arch Ophthalmol 1985;103:1796–806.
11. Van Leiden HA, Dekker JM, Moll AC, et al. Blood pressure, lipids, and obesity are associated with retinopathy: the Hoorn Study. Diabetes Care 2002;25(8): 1320–5.
12. Klein R, Moss SE, Klein BE. Is gross proteinuria a risk factor for the incidence of proliferative diabetic retinopathy? Ophthalmology 1993;100(8):1140–6.
13. Cruickshanks KJ, Ritter LL, Klein R, et al. The association of microalbuminuria with diabetic retinopathy. The Wisconsin Epidemiologic Study of Diabetic Retinopathy. Ophthalmology 1993;100(6):862–7.
14. Klein BE, Moss SE, Klein R. Effect of pregnancy on progression of diabetic retinopathy. Diabetes Care 1990;13(1):34–40.
15. Writing Team for the Diabetes Control and Complications Trial/Epidemiology of Diabetes Interventions and Complications Research Group. Effect of intensive therapy on the microvascular complications of type 1 diabetes mellitus. JAMA 2002;287(19):2563–9.
16. Chew EY, Ambrosius WT, Davis MD, et al, ACCORD Study Group, ACCORD Eye Study Group. Effects of medical therapies on retinopathy progression in type 2 diabetes. N Engl J Med 2010;363(3):233–44.
17. Keech A, Simes RJ, Barter P, et al. Effects of long-term fenofibrate therapy on cardiovascular events in 9795 people with type 2 diabetes mellitus (the FIELD study): randomised controlled trial. Lancet 2005;366(9500):1849–61.
18. Rodriguez-Fontal M, Kerrison JB, Alfaro DV, et al. Metabolic control and diabetic retinopathy. Curr Diabetes Rev 2009;5(1):3–7.
19. ADA. Standards of medical care in diabetes–2014. Diabetes Care 2014;37(Suppl 1):S14–80.

20. Mühlauser I, Sawicki P, Berger M. Cigarette smoking as a risk factor for macroproteinuria and proliferative retinopathy in type 1(insulin-dependent) diabetes. Diabetologia 1986;29:500–2.

21. Mühlhauser I, Bender R, Bott U, et al. Cigarette smoking and progression of retinopathy and nephropathy in type 1 diabetes. Diabet Med 1996;13:536–43.

22. Albert SG, Bernbaum M. Exercise for patients with diabetic retinopathy. Diabetes Care 1995;18(1):130–2.

23. The Diabetes Control and Complications Trial Research Group. Effect of pregnancy on microvascular complications in the diabetes control and complications trial. The Diabetes Control and Complications Trial Research Group. Diabetes Care 2000;23(8):1084–91.

24. Early treatment diabetic retinopathy study design and baseline patient characteristics. Ophthalmology 1991;98(5 Suppl):741–56.

25. Sivak-Callcott JA, O'Day DM, Gass JD, et al. Evidence-based recommendations for the diagnosis and treatment of neovascular glaucoma. Ophthalmology 2001; 108(10):1767–76.

26. Bressler NM, Edwards AR, Beck RW, et al. Exploratory analysis of the effect of intravitreal ranibizumab or triamcinolone on worsening of diabetic retinopathy in a randomized clinical trial. JAMA Ophthalmol 2013;131(8):1033–40.

27. Diabetic Retinopathy Clinical Research Network. Expanded 2-year follow-up of ranibizumab plus prompt or deferred laser or triamcinolone plus prompt laser for diabetic macular edema. Ophthalmology 2011;118(4):609–14.

28. Two-year course of visual acuity in severe proliferative diabetic retinopathy with conventional management. Diabetic Retinopathy Vitrectomy Study (DRVS) report #1. Ophthalmology 1985;92(4):492–502.

29. Diabetic Retinopathy Study Research Group. Photocoagulation treatment of proliferative diabetic retinopathy. Clinical applications of diabetic retinopathy study (DRS) findings, DRS report number 8. Ophthalmology 1981;88:583–600.

30. Canadian Ophthalmological Society. Canadian Ophthalmological Society evidence-based clinical practice guidelines for the management of diabetic retinopathy. Can J Ophthalmol 2012;47:S1–30.

Printed and bound by CPI Group (UK) Ltd, Croydon, CR0 4YY

18/10/2024

01775941-0004